W9-AEH-221

MATHEMATICS
FOR
HEALTH CAREERS

RT
68
.C38
1994

MATHEMATICS FOR HEALTH CAREERS

Carol Castellon, M.S. in Ed.

Deborah Baker, B.S. in Ed.

Carol Ann Stone, RN

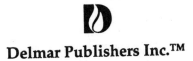

Delmar Publishers Inc.™

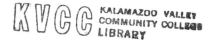

KVCC KALAMAZOO VALLEY
COMMUNITY COLLEGE
LIBRARY

MAY 1 4 1997

NOTICE TO READER

Publisher does not warrant or guarantee any of the products described herein or perform any independent analysis in connection with any of the product information contained herein. Publisher does not assume, and expressly disclaims, any obligation to obtain and include information other than that provided to it by the manufacturer.

The reader is expressly warned to consider and adopt all safety precautions that might be indicated by the activities described herein and to avoid all potential hazards. By following the instructions contained herein, the reader willingly assumes all risks in connection with such instructions.

The publisher makes no representations or warranties of any kind, including but not limited to, the warranties of fitness for particular purpose or merchantability, nor are any such representations implied with respect to the material set forth herein, and the publisher takes no responsibility with respect to such material. The publisher shall not be liable for any special, consequential or exemplary damages resulting, in whole or in part, from the readers' use of, or reliance upon, this material.

Cover design: Eva Ruutopõld

Delmar Staff:
Acquisitions Editor: Patricia E. Casey
Project Editor: Melissa A. Conan
Production Coordinator: Mary Ellen Black
Art and Design Coordinator: Mary E. Siener

For information, address

Delmar Publishers Inc.
3 Columbia Circle, Box 15015
Albany, NY 12212-5015

COPYRIGHT © 1994 BY DELMAR PUBLISHERS INC.

The trademark ITP is used under license.

All rights reserved. No part of this work covered by the copyright hereon may be reproduced or used in any form, or by any means—graphic, electronic, or mechanical, including photocopying, recording, taping, or information storage and retrieval systems—without written permission of the publisher.

Printed in the United States of America
Published simultaneously in Canada
by Nelson Canada,
a division of The Thomson Corporation
1 2 3 4 5 6 7 8 9 10   XXX   00 99 98 97 96 95 94

Library of Congress Cataloging-in-Publication Data
Castellon, Carol.
    Mathematics for health careers/by Carol Castellon, Deborah
Baker, Carol Ann Stone.
        p. cm.
    Includes index.
    ISBN 0–8273–5569-6
    1. Nursing—Mathematics.   2. Nursing—Mathematics—Problems,
exercises, etc.   3. Pharmaceutical arithmetic.   4. Pharmaceutical arithmetic—Problems, exercises, etc.
I. Baker, Deborah, 1948-   II. Stone, Carol Ann.   III. Title.
RT68.C38 1992
513′.024613—dc20
                                                                93-15623
                                                                    CIP

Mathematics for Health Careers is the product of many years of development and classroom testing at Parkland College (Champaign, Illinois). The book resulted from the expressed need by the nursing department to develop the mathematical skills of nursing students. We are especially concerned with developing comprehension and accuracy of word problems related to health careers.

The book is intended to help students who are beginning the study of nursing or plan to begin the study of nursing, to sharpen their mathematical skills before attempting a pharmaceutical course.

The book addresses three areas of mathematical literacy in health careers. Chapters 1–3 provide a review of arithmetic operations needed to calculate health-related problems.

Chapters 4–6 offer a comprehensive overview of the three systems of measurement used in health careers and conversion techniques. These systems are SI (metric system), the apothecaries' system, and the household system.

Chapters 7–8 present a variety of formulas and techniques needed to solve problems performed by health professionals. These include medication dosage problems of all levels of complexity, as well as solution preparation, IV administration, and pediatric dosage problems.

Chapter objectives give both the instructor and the student the intent and purpose of the chapter. The student will find many examples completely worked, followed by some "problems to try." The answers to these "problems to try" are found at the end of each exercise set. Each chapter of the book contains a wealth of word problems. All of the answers to the exercises as well as answers to the chapter tests are found in the back of the book.

Throughout the book, definitions are highlighted in single-line boxes, and rules are highlighted in double-line boxes.

The appendices contain a brief history of measurement, tables, and charts, and a comprehensive review of the entire book. The text is written so that calculators are not required to answer the questions, but instructors may opt to allow their use.

Abbreviation	Meaning	Abbreviation	Meaning
ROUTE		**FREQUENCY**	
IM	intramuscularly	q.h.	every hour
IV	intravenously	q.2h.	every two hours
IVPB	intravenous piggyback	q.3h.	every three hours
SC or SQ	subcutaneously	q.4h.	every four hours
PO or per os	by mouth	q.6h.	every six hours
OD	right eye	q.8h.	every eight hours
OS	left eye	q.12h.	every twelve hours
OU	both eyes	q.a.m.	every morning
NPO	nothing by mouth	q.p.m.	every evening
		q.h.s.	at bedtime
GENERAL		q.d.	every day
$\bar{a}$	before	q.o.d.	every other day
$\bar{p}$	after	b.i.d.	twice a day
$\bar{c}$	with	t.i.d.	three times a day
$\bar{s}$	without	q.i.d.	four times a day
$\bar{q}$	every	a.c.	before meals
gtt.	drop	p.c.	after meals
fld. or fl.	fluid	stat.	immediately
elix.	elixir	p.r.n.	when necessary
cap.	capsule	DC	discontinue
tab.	tablet		
susp.	suspension		
liq.	liquid		
N.S.	normal saline		
D/W	dextrose in water		
sol. or soln.	solution		
noc. or noct.	night		

*These are some of the abbreviations used in prescriptions and doctors' orders. You will have to know what the abbreviations mean in order to give a correct answer to some problems. If you are unfamiliar with these, memorize them immediately. This is only a partial list of common abbreviations; a more complete list can be found in pharmacy and nursing texts.

Table of Contents

We wish to extend our sincere thanks for the input or suggestions made by the following individuals: Dan Anderson, Debra Barnett, Barbara Buoy, Peter Folk, Mary Gallagher, Carol Larson, Lavern McFadden, Gian-Paolo Musumeci, Ricki Witz, and Debra Woods. In addition, we thank the following companies for permission to use their trademarks and for their assistance in preparing the word problems and exercises in this book.

The LifeCare Model 4 pump and nomogram chart (pp. 253 and 209, 267) courtesy of Abbott Laboratories. LIDOCAINE® (pp. 247, 249, 250, 259, 279), TRAN-XENE® (clorazepate dipotassium) (p. 28), QUELIDRINE® syrup (p. 111), NEMBUTAL® (pentobarbital sodium) (p. 161), and EES (erythromycin ethylsuccinate) (pp. 115, 144) are registered trademarks of Abbott Laboratories.

BUMEX® (bumetanide) (p. 28), VALIUM (diazepam) (pp. 28, 67, 177, 272), KLONOPIN® (clonazepam) (p. 202), TARACTAN® (chlorprothixene lactate and HCL) (p. 217), and GANTRISIN® (sulfisoxazole) (p. 204) are registered trademarks of Roche Laboratories, Hoffman-La Roche, Inc.

COUMADIN® (crystalline warfarin sodium) (pp. 27, 28) and NUBAIN® (nalbuphine hydrochloride) (p. 28) are registered trademarks of DuPont Merck Pharmaceutical Co.

ILOSONE® (erythromycin estolate) (pp. 165, 175, 200, 219, 275, 279) and KEFLEX® (cephalexin) (pp. 143, 165, 176, 199, 201, 204, 220) are registered trademarks of DISTA Products Company, Inc., a division of Eli Lilly and Co. KEFZOL (cefazolin sodium USP) (p. 184), CECLOR® (cefaclor USP) (pp. 203, 220), VANCOCIN® HCL (vancomycin hydrochloride) (p. 203), and ONCOVIN® (vincristine sulfate) (pp. 213, 220) are registered trademarks of Eli Lilly and Co.

LASIX® (furosemide) (p. 28) is a registered trademark of **Hoechst Aktiengesellschaft.**

SOLU-MEDROL® sterile powder (methylprednisolone sodium succinate) (p. 187) and CLEOCIN® PHOSPHATE sterile solution (clindamycin phosphate injection, USP) (p. 165), and DRAMAMINE® Tablets (dimenhidrinate) (p. 24) are registered trademarks of the Upjohn Co.

VISTARIL® (hydroxyzine pamoate) (pp. 165, 176, 178, 276) is a registered trademark of Pfizer Labs.

PREMARIN® (p. 65) and OMNIPEN® (ampicillin) (p. 202) are registered trademarks of Wyeth-Ayerst Laboratories.

DILAUDID® (p. 65) is a registered trademark of Knoll Pharmaceutical Co.

ZOVIRAX® (acyclovir) (pp. 214, 220) and LANOXIN® (p. 65) are registered trademarks of Burroughs Wellcome Co.

MAALOX® (pp. 92, 111) and TUSSAR® SF (p. 111) are registered trademarks of Rhône-Poulenc Rorer Pharmaceuticals Inc.

ADRIAMYCIN RDF® (doxorubicin hydrochloride) (p. 279) ADRIAMYCIN PFS® (doxorubicin hydrochloride) (pp. 213, 214, 220) are registered trademarks of Adria Laboratories.

KAON® Elixir (p. 115) is a registered trademark of Savage Laboratories, a division of Altana, Inc.

NITRO-BID® (p. 144) is used with permission of Marion Laboratories, Inc.

TUSSI-ORGANIDIN® (pp. 103, 114) is used with permission of Wallace Laboratories Division, Carter-Wallace, Inc., Canbury, New Jersey.

DILANTIN® (pp. 145, 161, 162) and CHLOROMYCETIN® (pp. 184, 202) are registered trademarks of the Warner-Lambert Co.

GARAMYCIN® (gentamicin sulfate) (p. 217) is a registered trademark of the Schering Corp.

MELLARIL® (thioridazine) (p. 217) is a registered trademark of and is used with the permission of the Sandoz Pharmaceuticals Corporation.

DEMEROL® (meperidine hydrochloride) (pp. 176, 177, 201, 219, 275), ISUPREL® (isoproterenol hydrochloride) (pp. 249, 250, 259), and ZEPHIRAN® Chloride (benzalkonium chloride) (pp. 197, 278) are registered trademarks of Sanofi Winthrop Pharmaceuticals.

PIPRACIL® (piperacillin sodium) (p. 187) is a registered trademark of Lederle Laboratories, a division of American Cyanamid Co.

MONOCID® (sterile cefonicid sodium [lyophilized]) (pp. 186, 276), TAZICEF® (ceftazidime) (pp. 188, 277), ANCEF (sterile cefazolin sodium [lyophilized]) (pp. 184, 188, 189, 190, 201, 219, 277, 279), and AMOXIL® (pp. 103, 279) are registered trademarks of SmithKline Beecham.

CEFIZOX® (p. 189) is a registered trademark of Fujisawa Pharmaceuticals.

Children's PANADOL® (acetaminophen) (pp. 203, 219) is a registered trademark of Sterling Winthrop Inc., New York, N.Y.

ELIXOPHYLLIN® (p. 203) is a registered trademark of Forest Pharmaceuticals, Inc.

PRONESTYL® (p. 250) is a registered trademark of Apothecon, a subsidiary of Bristol-Myers Squibb Co.

DOPAMINE® (pp. 249, 250, 279) is a registered trademark of Astra Pharmaceutical Products, Inc.

Chapter 1

Fractions

This chapter is a review of fractions. When you complete this chapter you should be able to:

a. Add, subtract, multiply, and divide fractions.
b. Identify proper, improper, and mixed fractions.
c. Reduce fractions to lowest terms.
d. Use fractions in working simple word problems.

1.1 *Defining Terms*

FRACTION - tells what part of a whole.
NUMERATOR - is the top number in a fraction and tells how many parts are being considered.
DENOMINATOR - is the bottom number in a fraction and tells how many parts the whole is divided into.

Since division by zero is undefined, the denominator of a fraction can never be zero. For example, $\frac{3}{0}$ is not a valid fraction.

What fraction will represent the shaded area in the rectangle below? The rectangle is divided into 8 equal parts, so the denominator is 8. There are 3 squares shaded, so the numerator is 3.

Therefore the shaded area is represented by the fraction $\frac{3}{8}$.

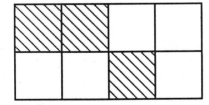

Problems to try. Answers to these problems appear at the end of 1.1 exercises.

a. What fractional part of the previous rectangle is not shaded?_____

b. This circle is divided into how many parts?_____

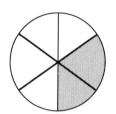

How many parts are shaded?_____

What fraction of the circle is shaded?_____

The fraction discussed so far is called a proper fraction.

PROPER FRACTION - the numerator is always less than the denominator and the value of the fraction is less than 1.

Examples: $\dfrac{7}{12}$ $\dfrac{140}{143}$ $\dfrac{3}{7}$ $\dfrac{12}{17}$

Another kind of fraction is an improper fraction.

IMPROPER FRACTION - the numerator is equal to or greater than the denominator and the value of the fraction is equal to or greater than 1.

Examples: $\dfrac{7}{7}$ $\dfrac{12}{7}$ $\dfrac{13}{13}$ $\dfrac{120}{113}$

Problems to try.

c. This circle is divided into how many parts?_____

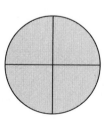

How many parts are shaded?_____

Represent the shaded area as a fraction._____

Is this fraction proper or improper?_____

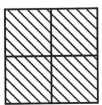 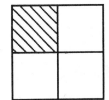

Above are two squares. Each is divided into four parts, so the denominator is 4. Five parts are shaded, so the numerator is 5. The fraction $\frac{5}{4}$ represents the shaded parts of these two squares. $\frac{5}{4}$ is an improper fraction.

Problems to try.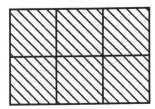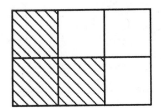

d. Each rectangle is divided into how many parts?_____

How many parts are shaded?_____

Represent the shaded area as a fraction._____

Is this fraction proper or improper?_____

MIXED NUMBER - consists of a whole number and a proper fraction. A mixed number is always greater than one.

Examples: $1\frac{3}{4}$ $12\frac{7}{8}$ $4\frac{11}{12}$

1.1 Exercises

Express the shaded area as a fraction.

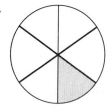 1.   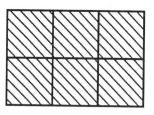 2.   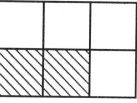   1. ___

   2. ___

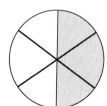 3.   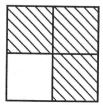 4.   3. ___

   4. ___

Determine if these fractions are proper, improper, or mixed.

5. $\frac{3}{7}$ _____   6. $\frac{12}{5}$ _____

7. $\frac{8}{9}$ _____   8. $1\frac{3}{5}$ _____

9. $12\frac{4}{11}$ _____   10. $\frac{15}{4}$ _____

11. $\frac{27}{8}$ _____   12. $\frac{1}{3}$ _____

13.   Carol gave 4 tablets out of a pack containing 16. What fractional part of the medication has she given?

14.   Pam's cough syrup bottle contained 12 ounces. Only 4 ounces are left. What fractional part was given?

Answers to Problems to try.

a. $\frac{5}{8}$ b. 6, 2, $\frac{2}{6}$ c. 4, 4, $\frac{4}{4}$, improper   d. 6, 9, $\frac{9}{6}$, improper

---

1.2   Changing the Form of the Fraction

It is necessary to change the form of a fraction before adding, subtracting, multiplying, or dividing fractions. The line separating the numerator and denominator of a fraction is called a division bar.

Example: $\frac{7}{8}$ can be read as 7 divided by 8 and written as $8\overline{)7}$

CHANGING AN IMPROPER FRACTION TO A MIXED NUMBER:
1.   **divide the numerator by the denominator;**
2.   **the quotient is the whole number;**
3.   **the remainder, if any, is the numerator of the fractional part of the mixed number;**
4.   **the denominator of this fractional part is the same as the original denominator.**

Example: Change $\frac{25}{8}$ to a mixed number.

$$
\begin{array}{r}
3 \\
\text{denominator } 8 \,\overline{)25} \\
24 \\
\hline
1
\end{array}
\quad
\begin{array}{l}
\text{whole number} \\
\\
\\
\text{numerator}
\end{array}
\qquad = 3\frac{1}{8}
$$

Problems to try. Answers to these problems appear at the end of 1.2 exercises.

a. Change $\frac{22}{5}$ to a mixed number.

$$\begin{array}{r} 4 \quad \text{whole number} \qquad =\underline{\hspace{2cm}} \\ \text{denominator } 5\,\overline{)\,22} \\ \underline{20} \\ 2 \quad \text{numerator} \end{array}$$

b. Change $\frac{18}{3}$ to a mixed number. $=\underline{\hspace{2cm}}$

c. Change $\frac{29}{4}$ to a mixed number. $=\underline{\hspace{2cm}}$

CHANGE A MIXED NUMBER TO AN IMPROPER FRACTION:
1. multiply the whole number times the denominator of the fractional part of the mixed number;
2. add this to the numerator of the fractional part;
3. place this sum over the original denominator.

Example: Change $2\frac{3}{5}$ to an improper fraction.

$$2 \times 5 = 10 \qquad 10 + 3 = 13 \qquad \frac{13}{5}$$

Example: Change $12\frac{2}{3}$ to an improper fraction.

$$12 \times 3 = 36 \qquad 36 + 2 = 38 \qquad \frac{38}{3}$$

Problems to try.

d. Change $9\frac{7}{8}$ to an improper fraction.

$$9 \times 8 = \underline{\hspace{0.7cm}} \quad \underline{\hspace{0.7cm}} + \underline{\hspace{0.7cm}} = \underline{\hspace{0.7cm}} \qquad \underline{\hspace{2cm}}$$

e. Change $11\frac{3}{4}$ to an improper fraction. $\underline{\hspace{2.5cm}}$

EQUIVALENT FRACTIONS have the same value.

Examples: $\frac{1}{2} = \frac{2}{4}$ $\frac{1}{3} = \frac{2}{6}$ $\frac{4}{10} = \frac{2}{5}$

An equivalent fraction can be found by multiplying or dividing the numerator and the denominator by the same non-zero number.

Example: Find an equivalent fraction for $\frac{3}{4}$.

$$\frac{3 \times 2}{4 \times 2} = \frac{6}{8} \qquad \frac{3 \times 3}{4 \times 3} = \frac{9}{12} \qquad \frac{3 \times 4}{4 \times 4} = \frac{12}{16}$$

An infinite amount of equivalent numbers can be found using this method.

Example: Change the fraction $\frac{3}{4}$ to an equivalent fraction with a denominator of 20. What would the numerator be?

$$\frac{3}{4} = \frac{?}{20} \qquad \text{What times 4 gives 20? } (20 \div 4 = 5)$$

$$\frac{3 \times 5}{4 \times 5} = \frac{15}{20} \quad \text{Now multiply the same number times the numerator.}$$

Problems to try. Fill in the blanks.

f. $\frac{7 \times}{8 \times} \underline{} = \frac{}{16}$

g. $\frac{11 \times}{5 \times} \underline{} = \frac{}{15}$

Reducing is another way to find an equivalent fraction.

To reduce fractions divide the numerator and the denominator by the same number.

Example: Reduce $\frac{12}{15}$ to lowest terms.

$$\frac{12 \div 3}{15 \div 3} = \frac{4}{5}$$

Example: The fraction $\frac{54}{36}$ can be reduced several different ways.

$$\frac{54}{36} \div \frac{2}{2} = \frac{27}{18} \div \frac{3}{3} = \frac{9}{6} \div \frac{3}{3} = \frac{3}{2} \quad \text{or} \quad \frac{54}{36} \div \frac{9}{9} = \frac{6}{4} \div \frac{2}{2} = \frac{3}{2}$$

Reducing a fraction to **lowest terms** means that the numerator and denominator cannot be divided by the same number. In the preceding example, $\frac{3}{2}$ is in lowest terms because there is no number that will divide evenly into both 3 and 2.

Problems to try. Reduce these fractions to lowest terms.

h. $\frac{63}{105} =$ _____   i. $\frac{5}{13} =$ _____

DIVISIBILITY TESTS:
1. **If a number is even, it is divisible by 2.**
2. **If the sum of the digits of a number are divisible by 3, then the number is divisible by 3.**
3. **If a number ends in five or zero, it is divisible by 5.**
4. **If a number ends in zero, it is divisible by 10.**

All answers should be **simplified**; that is, reduced to lowest terms and put in the form of proper fractions or mixed numbers, unless otherwise stated.

Example: Simplify $\frac{24}{16}$

$$\frac{24}{16} \div \frac{8}{8} = \frac{3}{2} = 1\frac{1}{2} \quad \text{or} \quad \frac{24}{16} = 1\frac{8}{16} = 1\frac{1}{2}$$

Example: Simplify $2\frac{5}{3}$ This is not a mixed number in proper form because the fractional part is an improper fraction.

$2 + \frac{5}{3}$ separate the whole number from the fraction

$2 + 1\frac{2}{3}$ change $\frac{5}{3}$ to a mixed number

$3\frac{2}{3}$ then add

Problems to try. Simplify these fractions.

j. $\frac{42}{30}$ = _____

k. $7\frac{12}{5}$ = _____

Change a whole number to a fraction by placing the number over 1.

Examples: $6 = \frac{6}{1}$ $12 = \frac{12}{1}$ $155 = \frac{155}{1}$

Change 1 to a fraction by placing any number over itself.

Examples: $1 = \frac{12}{12} = \frac{145}{145} = \frac{3}{3} = \frac{6}{6} = \frac{54}{54} = \frac{15}{15}$, etc.

1.2   Exercises

Change to a mixed number:

1. $\frac{13}{2}$ _____

2. $\frac{16}{7}$ _____

3. $\frac{17}{4}$ _____

4. $\frac{35}{3}$ _____

5. $\frac{68}{9}$ _____

6. $\frac{39}{16}$ _____

7. $\frac{21}{8}$ _____

8. $\frac{23}{17}$ _____

Change to an improper fraction:

9. $6\frac{3}{4}$ _____

10. $5\frac{1}{17}$ _____

11. $7\frac{3}{11}$ _____

12. $5\frac{2}{3}$ _____

13. $6\frac{2}{9}$ _____

14. 9 _____

15. $11\frac{3}{5}$ _____

16. $21\frac{3}{4}$ _____

Fill in the blank:

17. $\frac{2}{3} = \frac{}{15}$

18. $\frac{5}{8} = \frac{}{24}$

19. $\frac{7}{6} = \frac{}{24}$

20. $\frac{6}{7} = \frac{}{28}$

21. $\frac{1}{4} = \frac{}{36}$

22. $\frac{12}{15} = \frac{}{60}$

Reduce to lowest terms:

23. $\frac{12}{20}$ _____

24. $\frac{10}{90}$ _____

25. $\frac{26}{39}$ _____

26. $\frac{36}{48}$ _____

27. $\frac{42}{36}$ _____

28. $\frac{35}{50}$ _____

29. $\frac{48}{120}$ _____

30. $\frac{30}{42}$ _____

Simplify:

31. $\frac{42}{8}$ _____

32. $\frac{34}{16}$ _____

33. $\frac{35}{5}$ _____   34. $\frac{50}{12}$ _____

35. $3\frac{9}{6}$ _____   36. $7\frac{12}{5}$ _____

37. $12\frac{9}{3}$ _____   38. $1\frac{7}{2}$ _____

Answers to Problems to try.

a. $4\frac{2}{5}$ b. 6   c. $7\frac{1}{4}$ d. $\frac{79}{8}$ e. $\frac{47}{4}$ f. 14   g. 33   h. $\frac{3}{5}$

i. $\frac{5}{13}$ j. $1\frac{2}{5}$ k. $9\frac{2}{5}$

1.3   Adding and Subtracting Fractions

Before adding or subtracting fractions, you must first find a common denominator. One way to find a common denominator is by multiplying the denominators together, but this may give a denominator that is large and hard to work with. There is more chance for errors with a larger number than with a smaller one. Instead, find the **smallest common denominator**.

> **COMMON DENOMINATOR**   is the smallest multiple of the original denominators.

> **TO FIND THE MULTIPLE OF A NUMBER:**
> 1. multiply the number times one;
> 2. multiply the number times 2;
> 3. multiply the number times 3;
> 4. etc.

Example: Find the multiples of 5.

$5 \times 1 = 5$

$5 \times 2 = 10$

$5 \times 3 = 15$

$5 \times 4 = 20$ etc.

The multiples of 5 are: 5   10   15   20   25   30   35, etc.

TO FIND A COMMON DENOMINATOR:
  1. **list the multiples of each denominator;**
  2. **find the smallest common multiple.**

Example: Find a common denominator for 6 and 9.

Multiples of 6:   6   12   18   24   30   36
Multiples of 9:   9   18   27   36   45   54

The smallest common multiple is 18, so 18 is the common denominator.

Example: Find a common denominator for 8 and 6:

Multiples of 6:   6   12   18   24   30
Multiples of 8:   8   16   24

24 is the first common multiple, so 24 is the common denominator.

Example: Find a common denominator for 10 and 3:

Multiples of 3:   3   6   9   12   15   18   21   24   27   30
Multiples of 10:   10   20   30

30 is the first common multiple, so 30 is the common denominator.

Problems to try. Answers to these problems appear at the end of 1.3 exercises.

a. Find a common denominator for 5 and 8:   _____

b. Find a common denominator for 2, 3 and 5:   _____

TO ADD FRACTIONS:
1. find a common denominator;
2. add the numerators;
3. place this sum over the common denominator;
4. simplify.

Example: $\frac{2}{7} + \frac{3}{7} = \frac{2+3}{7} = \frac{5}{7}$

Example: $\frac{3}{4} + \frac{3}{8} =$ The common denominator is 8.

Change $\frac{3}{4}$ to $\frac{?}{8} = \frac{3 \times 2}{4 \times 2} = \frac{6}{8}$

$\frac{6}{8} + \frac{3}{8} = \frac{9}{8} = 1\frac{1}{8}$

Example: $\frac{3}{5} + \frac{2}{3} =$ The common denominator is 15.

$\frac{3}{5} = \frac{9}{15}$ and $\frac{2}{3} = \frac{10}{15}$

$\frac{9}{15} + \frac{10}{15} = \frac{19}{15} = 1\frac{4}{15}$

Problems to try.

c. $\frac{1}{2} + \frac{1}{3} =$ The common denominator is _____

$\frac{1}{2} =$ _____ $\frac{1}{3} =$ _____

The answer is _____

d. $\frac{3}{10} + \frac{1}{3} =$ _____

TO ADD MIXED NUMBERS:
1. **find a common denominator;**
2. **add the whole numbers;**
3. **add the fractional parts;**
4. **simplify.**

Examples:

$$1\frac{1}{2} = 1\frac{4}{8}$$
$$+2\frac{5}{8} = 2\frac{5}{8}$$
$$\overline{\qquad}$$
$$3\frac{9}{8} = 4\frac{1}{8}$$

$$12$$
$$+ 7\frac{3}{5}$$
$$\overline{\qquad}$$
$$19\frac{3}{5}$$

Problems to try.

e.
$$2\frac{1}{6}$$
$$\frac{3}{4}$$
$$+1\frac{3}{8}$$
$$\overline{\qquad}$$

f.
$$3\frac{5}{6}$$
$$+4\frac{1}{4}$$
$$\overline{\qquad}$$

TO SUBTRACT FRACTIONS:
1. **find a common denominator;**
2. **subtract the numerators;**
3. **place this number over the common denominator;**
4. **simplify.**

Example: $\dfrac{5}{6} - \dfrac{2}{6} = \dfrac{5-2}{6} = \dfrac{3}{6} = \dfrac{1}{2}$

Example: $\dfrac{7}{8} - \dfrac{1}{2} =$ The common denominator is 8.

Change $\dfrac{1}{2}$ to $\dfrac{4}{8}$

$\dfrac{7}{8} - \dfrac{4}{8} = \dfrac{3}{8}$

Problems to try.

g. $\dfrac{4}{5} - \dfrac{2}{3} =$ _____

h. $\dfrac{15}{12} - \dfrac{1}{3} =$ _____

TO SUBTRACT MIXED NUMBERS:
1. change each fractional part to a common denominator;
2a. if the fraction being subtracted is smaller, subtract the fractional parts;
2b. if the fraction being subtracted is larger, borrow 1 from the whole number and add it to the fractional part; then subtract the fractional parts;
3. subtract the whole numbers;
4. simplify.

Example: $9\frac{3}{4} - 7\frac{1}{2} =$ Find a common denominator and change each fractional part.

Write the numbers in vertical order for ease of operation.

$$\begin{array}{l} 9\frac{3}{4} = 9\frac{3}{4} \\ -7\frac{1}{2} = 7\frac{2}{4} \\ \hline \quad\;\; 2\frac{1}{4} \end{array}$$

Subtract the fractions.

Subtract the whole numbers.

Example: $12\frac{1}{6} - 4\frac{1}{2} =$ Find the common denominator and change.

$$\begin{array}{l} 12\frac{1}{6} = 12\frac{1}{6} \\ -4\frac{1}{2} = \;\;4\frac{3}{6} \\ \hline \end{array}$$

$\frac{3}{6}$ is larger than $\frac{1}{6}$ so you must borrow.

To borrow, change $12\frac{1}{6}$.

$$12\frac{1}{6} = 12 + \frac{1}{6} = 11 + 1 + \frac{1}{6} = 11 + \frac{6}{6} + \frac{1}{6} = 11 + \frac{7}{6} = 11\frac{7}{6}$$

$$\begin{array}{l} 12\frac{1}{6} = 11\frac{7}{6} \\ -4\frac{3}{6} = \;\;4\frac{3}{6} \\ \hline \quad\quad\;\; 7\frac{4}{6} = 7\frac{2}{3} \end{array}$$

Subtract the fractions, then subtract the whole numbers and simplify.

Example:

$$\begin{array}{l} 8 \\ -2\frac{5}{8} \\ \hline \end{array}$$

$8 = 7 + 1 = 7 + \frac{8}{8} = 7\frac{8}{8}$

Borrow and subtract.

$$\begin{array}{l} 7\frac{8}{8} \\ -2\frac{5}{8} \\ \hline \;\; 5\frac{3}{8} \end{array}$$

Problems to try.

i. $4\frac{7}{8} - 1\frac{3}{4} =$ _____

j. $2\frac{1}{12} - 1\frac{1}{8} =$ _____

1.3 Exercises

Perform the indicated operations and simplify.

1. $\frac{3}{4} + \frac{5}{6}$ _____

2. $\frac{1}{3} + \frac{3}{4}$ _____

3. $\frac{7}{8} + \frac{3}{10}$ _____

4. $\frac{9}{8} + \frac{5}{6}$ _____

5. $\frac{3}{4} + \frac{1}{3} + \frac{5}{8}$ _____

6. $\frac{3}{10} + \frac{7}{15} + \frac{1}{5}$ _____

7. $\frac{1}{2} + \frac{1}{3} + \frac{1}{4}$ _____

8. $9 + \frac{2}{3}$ _____

9. $2\frac{3}{4} + 12\frac{7}{8}$ _____

10. $8\frac{3}{4} + 9\frac{5}{6}$ _____

11. $2\frac{1}{3} + 5\frac{3}{5}$ _____

12. $\frac{3}{8} + 4\frac{1}{6}$ _____

13. $3\frac{5}{6} + 2\frac{3}{4}$ _____

14. $6 + 1\frac{3}{5} + 2\frac{3}{10}$ _____

15. $7\frac{1}{8} + \frac{2}{3} + 4$ _____

16. $\frac{3}{4} - \frac{3}{5}$ _____

17. $\frac{5}{8} - \frac{3}{6}$ _____

18. $\frac{5}{6} - \frac{3}{4}$ _____

19. $\frac{2}{3} - \frac{2}{5}$ _____

20. $\frac{7}{9} - \frac{1}{6}$ _____

21. $\frac{6}{7} - \frac{2}{3}$ _____

22. $18 - 6\frac{2}{5}$ _____

23. $4\frac{1}{2} - 2\frac{3}{7}$ _____

24. $4\frac{7}{8} - 1\frac{3}{4}$ _____

25. $6\frac{5}{12} - 4\frac{5}{8}$ _____

26. $6 - 1\frac{1}{2}$ _____

27. $11\frac{1}{8} - 6\frac{1}{6}$ _____

28. Joe walked several times during the week. He walked $\frac{1}{3}$ mile, $\frac{7}{12}$ mile, and $\frac{5}{6}$ mile. How many miles did he walk altogether?

29. Nancy started dieting and lost $9\frac{1}{2}$ lbs. the first week. The second week she gained $\frac{1}{4}$ of a lb. The third week she lost $2\frac{3}{4}$ lbs., and the fourth week she lost $1\frac{1}{2}$ lbs. How many pounds had she lost at the end of the month?

Answers to Problems to try.

a. 40   b. 30   c. 6, $\frac{3}{6}$, $\frac{2}{6}$, $\frac{5}{6}$ d. $\frac{19}{30}$ e. $4\frac{7}{24}$ f. $8\frac{1}{12}$ g. $\frac{2}{15}$

h. $\frac{11}{12}$ i. $3\frac{1}{8}$ j. $\frac{23}{24}$

1.4 Multiplying and Dividing Fractions

> **TO MULTIPLY FRACTIONS:**
>   1. change mixed numbers to improper fractions;
>   2. try to cancel one numerator and one denominator;
>   3. multiply numerators;
>   4. multiply denominators;
>   5. simplify.

Example: $\dfrac{4}{9} \times \dfrac{15}{14}$

$$\dfrac{\overset{2}{\cancel{4}}}{\underset{3}{\cancel{9}}} \times \dfrac{\overset{5}{\cancel{15}}}{\underset{7}{\cancel{14}}}$$ Cancel a 2 out of 4 and 14, and 3 out of 9 and 15.

$$\dfrac{2 \times 5}{3 \times 7} = \dfrac{10}{21}$$ Multiply numerators and denominators.

Example: $6 \times \dfrac{9}{30} =$

$$\dfrac{6}{1} \times \dfrac{9}{30}$$ Change 6 to a fraction by putting it over 1.

$$\dfrac{\overset{1}{\cancel{6}}}{1} \times \dfrac{9}{\underset{5}{\cancel{30}}}$$ Cancel 6 out of 6 and 30.

$$\dfrac{1 \times 9}{1 \times 5} = \dfrac{9}{5}$$ Multiply numerators and denominators.

$$\dfrac{9}{5} = 1\dfrac{4}{5}$$ Simplify.

Example: $5\frac{1}{4} \times 2\frac{2}{7} =$

$\frac{21}{4} \times \frac{16}{7}$ Change to improper fractions.

$\frac{\overset{3}{\cancel{21}}}{\underset{1}{\cancel{4}}} \times \frac{\overset{4}{\cancel{16}}}{\underset{1}{\cancel{7}}}$ Cancel.

$\frac{3 \times 4}{1 \times 1} = \frac{12}{1} = 12$ Multiply and simplify.

Problems to try. Answers to these problems appear at the end of 1.4 exercises.

a. $\frac{4}{10} \times \frac{6}{8} =$ _____

b. $25 \times 1\frac{1}{5} =$ _____

c. $2\frac{1}{7} \times 2\frac{4}{5} =$ _____

TO DIVIDE FRACTIONS:
1.   **change mixed numbers to improper fractions;**
2.   **invert the divisor (second number), and change the sign to multiplication;**
3.   **try to cancel one numerator and one denominator;**
4.   **multiply and simplify.**

Example: $\frac{5}{8} \div \frac{1}{2} =$

$\frac{5}{8} \times \frac{2}{1}$ Invert the second number and change to multiplication.

$\frac{5}{\underset{4}{\cancel{8}}} \times \frac{\overset{1}{\cancel{2}}}{1}$ Cancel, multiply and simplify.

$\frac{5 \times 1}{4 \times 1} = \frac{5}{4} = 1\frac{1}{4}$

Example: $1\frac{5}{7} \div \frac{3}{4} =$

$\frac{12}{7} \times \frac{4}{3}$ Change to improper fraction, invert the divisor, and change to multiplication.

$\frac{\overset{4}{\cancel{12}}}{7} \times \frac{4}{\underset{1}{\cancel{3}}}$ Cancel, multiply and simplify.

$\frac{4 \times 4}{7 \times 1} = \frac{16}{7} = 2\frac{2}{7}$

Example: $\frac{4}{9} \div 2 =$

$\frac{4}{9} \div \frac{2}{1} = \frac{4}{9} \times \frac{1}{2} = \frac{\overset{2}{\cancel{4}}}{9} \times \frac{1}{\underset{1}{\cancel{2}}} = \frac{2 \times 1}{9 \times 1} = \frac{2}{9}$

Example: $2\frac{1}{6} \div 3\frac{1}{4} =$

$\frac{13}{6} \div \frac{13}{4} = \frac{13}{6} \times \frac{4}{13} = \frac{\overset{1}{\cancel{13}}}{\underset{3}{\cancel{6}}} \times \frac{\overset{2}{\cancel{4}}}{\underset{1}{\cancel{13}}} = \frac{1 \times 2}{3 \times 1} = \frac{2}{3}$

Problems to try.

d. $\frac{3}{9} \div 1\frac{1}{3} =$ _____

e. $6 \div \frac{1}{4} =$ _____

f. $3\frac{1}{3} \div 5\frac{1}{2} =$ _____

COMPLEX FRACTION - the numerator, the denominator, or both are proper, improper, or mixed fractions.

Complex fractions can be simplified by division.

Example: $\frac{\frac{1}{5}}{7} = \frac{1}{5} \div 7 = \frac{1}{5} \div \frac{7}{1} = \frac{11}{5} \times \frac{1}{7} = \frac{1 \times 1}{5 \times 7} = \frac{1}{35}$

Example: $\frac{1\frac{2}{3}}{\frac{7}{9}} = \frac{5}{3} \div \frac{7}{9} = \frac{5}{\underset{1}{\cancel{3}}} \times \frac{\overset{3}{\cancel{9}}}{7} = \frac{5 \times 3}{1 \times 7} = \frac{15}{7} = 2\frac{1}{7}$

Perform the indicated operations and simplify.

1. $\dfrac{2}{3} \times \dfrac{1}{3}$ _____

2. $\dfrac{3}{5} \times \dfrac{5}{8}$ _____

3. $\dfrac{6}{25} \times \dfrac{10}{21}$ _____

4. $6\dfrac{1}{2} \times \dfrac{4}{13}$ _____

5. $6 \times \dfrac{4}{9}$ _____

6. $15 \times \dfrac{4}{35}$ _____

7. $1\dfrac{5}{7} \times \dfrac{1}{6}$ _____

8. $1\dfrac{3}{4} \times \dfrac{4}{5}$ _____

9. $\dfrac{3}{8} \times \dfrac{4}{5} \times \dfrac{15}{9}$ _____

10. $\dfrac{5}{8} \times 2\dfrac{1}{2}$ _____

11. $\dfrac{3}{7} \times 3\dfrac{1}{9}$ _____

12. $1\dfrac{1}{3} \times 1\dfrac{1}{2}$ _____

13. $12\dfrac{1}{2} \div \dfrac{5}{8}$ _____

14. $2\dfrac{1}{6} \div 2\dfrac{3}{5}$ _____

15. $5\dfrac{1}{3} \div 2\dfrac{2}{3}$ _____

16. $\dfrac{4}{9} \div 6$ _____

17. $3\dfrac{3}{5} \div \dfrac{6}{25}$ _____

18. $10\dfrac{2}{5} \div \dfrac{13}{15}$ _____

19. $6 \div 2\dfrac{1}{7}$ _____

20. $\dfrac{4}{9} \div 36$ _____

21. $3\frac{3}{4} \div 5\frac{5}{6}$ _____

22. $\dfrac{6\frac{4}{5}}{1\frac{7}{10}}$ _____

23. $\dfrac{6\frac{1}{5}}{6\frac{1}{5}}$ _____

24. $\dfrac{2\frac{1}{2}}{1\frac{3}{4}}$ _____

25. If the nurse gives $1\frac{1}{2}$ tablets each day for 7 days, how many tablets does she give all together?

26. If a medication bubble pack contains 30 tablets and the doctor has ordered $1\frac{1}{2}$ tablets q.i.d. How many days will the medication last?

Answers to Problems to try.

a. $\frac{3}{10}$ b. 30   c. 6   d. $\frac{1}{4}$ e. 24   f. $\frac{20}{33}$

1.5   Word Problems

```
REMEMBER
    Total medication = Amount per tablet × Number of tablets
    Number of tablets = Total medication ÷ Amt. per tablet
```

Read the problem to determine what information is given and what must be found.

Look for words that give a hint as to whether you should add, subtract, multiply or divide to get the answer.

When you get the answer, go back and read the problem to see if your answer makes sense.

Example: You give a patient three tablets from a bottle labeled $\frac{3}{4}$ grain each. How much medication has he received?

Number of tablets = 3

Amount per tablet = $\frac{3}{4}$ grain

Total medication = $3 \times \frac{3}{4} = \frac{9}{4} = 2\frac{1}{4}$ grain

Example: To give 75 mg of medication from 150 mg tablets, how may tablets should be given?

Total medication = 75 mg

Amount per tablet = 150 mg

Number of tablets = $75 \div 150 = \frac{1}{2}$ tablet

Keep in mind that a half of a tablet can only be given if the tablet is scored in halves. If the tablet is unscored, it cannot be broken in half. If you calculate the dose to be half of a tablet and the tablet is unscored, look for a different strength tablet or consult the doctor or pharmacist. Tablets are rarely scored in fourths.

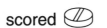

scored   unscored

1.5   Exercises

1. Pam has taken 6 tablets out of a bottle containing 30 tablets. What fractional part of the total tablets available has she taken?

2. John has a bottle containing 24 caplets. Of these, he has taken 8. What fractional part of the total caplets available is left in the bottle?

3. The pharmacy has 57 capsules of a new medication. They must make up sample packets containing 6 capsules each. How many complete sample packets can they make?

4. If a bottle of medicine holds $7\frac{1}{2}$ oz. and the patient takes $\frac{1}{5}$ of the bottle, how many ounces of medicine are left in the bottle?

5. If a patient receives $\frac{1}{2}$ of a $\frac{1}{4}$-grain morphine sulfate tablet, how much of the medication did the patient receive?

6. To give 50 mg of ascorbic acid from 100 mg tablets, how many tablets should be given?

7. To give 50 mg of ascorbic acid from 200 mg tablets, how many tablets should be used?

8. A nurse used three 4-grain potassium permanganate tablets in the preparation of a medication. How much potassium permanganate did she use?

9. A patient is given one 15 mg phenobarbital tablet t.i.d. How many milligrams of phenobarbital did the patient receive in one day?

10. The doctor orders 75 mg of DRAMAMINE® Tablets (dimenhidrinate). If the tablets on hand contain 50 mg per tablet, how many tablets should the nurse give?

11. If a patient is given $\frac{1}{2}$ of a 5-grain aspirin tablet, how many grains did the patient receive?

12. If you used $\frac{1}{2}$ of a 10-grain tablet, how many grains did you use?

13. If a patient is to be given $\frac{1}{2}$ grain of medication from $\frac{1}{4}$-grain tablets, how many tablets would be given?

14. To give 625 mg of ascorbic acid from 250 mg tablets, how many tablets would you use?

15. Bob drank $\frac{4}{9}$ of his water on Monday, $\frac{1}{3}$ of his water on Tuesday, and $\frac{1}{6}$ of his water on Wednesday. What fractional part of his water did he drink altogether?

16. In one week, Linda jogged $\frac{1}{4}$ mile, $\frac{5}{12}$ mile, and $\frac{5}{6}$ mile. How many miles did she jog altogether?

17. Jack went on a diet. He started out weighing $187\frac{1}{2}$ lbs. The first week he lost $10\frac{1}{4}$ lbs.; the second week he lost $9\frac{3}{8}$ lbs.; the third week he lost $5\frac{3}{4}$ lbs.; and the fourth week he lost $1\frac{1}{2}$ lbs. What did he weigh at the end of the fourth week?

18. Mary went on a diet. She started out weighing $145\frac{3}{4}$ lbs. The first week she lost $6\frac{1}{4}$ lbs.; the second week she lost $4\frac{3}{8}$ lbs.; the third week she lost $1\frac{5}{8}$ lbs.; and the fourth week she gained $\frac{1}{2}$ lb. What did she weigh at the end of the fourth week?

19. A patient receives 3 gr., $1\frac{1}{4}$ gr., $2\frac{1}{8}$ gr. and $\frac{1}{2}$ gr. of medication during the day. How many grains of medication has he taken all day?

20. A patient is to receive $\frac{3}{4}$ oz. q.3h. How much medication would you order for a 3 day supply?

21. You gave $\frac{3}{4}$ oz. from a bottle containing $2\frac{1}{2}$ oz. How much is left in the bottle?

22. You give a patient $1\frac{1}{2}$ oz. of a medicine q.3h. After one day, how much medicine is left in a 20 ounce bottle?

23. A patient is to receive $\frac{1}{2}$ gr. q.8h. How much medication will she receive in a 2-day period?

24. Dan jogged $15\frac{3}{4}$ miles and Frank jogged $12\frac{5}{6}$ miles. How many more miles did Dan jog than Frank?

Space Provided for Student Work

Chapter 1 Test

Perform the indicated operations and simplify.

1. $\dfrac{5}{8} + \dfrac{7}{10}$ _____

2. $3\dfrac{1}{3} + 4\dfrac{3}{5}$ _____

3. $\dfrac{7}{8} - \dfrac{3}{6}$ _____

4. $8 - 2\dfrac{4}{7}$ _____

5. $4\dfrac{3}{8} - 1\dfrac{3}{4}$ _____

6. $7 \times \dfrac{4}{21}$ _____

7. $16\dfrac{1}{2} \times 1\dfrac{5}{11}$ _____

8. $1\dfrac{1}{15} \div 3\dfrac{1}{5}$ _____

9. $\dfrac{5\frac{1}{3}}{2\frac{2}{3}}$ _____

10. If John is to take 10 mg of COUMADIN ® (crystalline warfarin sodium) daily, how many $2\dfrac{1}{2}$ mg tablets should he take?

11. In giving a patient her medication, $\dfrac{4}{5}$ of a 10 cc vial was used. How many cc's will be discarded?

12. If a patient receives 5 grains, $7\dfrac{1}{2}$ grains and $\dfrac{3}{8}$ grain of medication, how many total grains has he received?

13. You give a patient two tablets from a bottle labeled $\frac{3}{4}$ grains each. How many grains has he received?

14. NUBAIN® (nalbuphine hydrochloride) is available in a multiple dose vial labeled: 10 ml (10 mg per ml). How many milligrams would be in half of the vial?

15. If, over the course of a week, the doctor changed John's dose of COUMADIN® (crystalline warfarin sodium) daily, and he received 2 mg, $2\frac{1}{2}$ mg, 5 mg, $7\frac{1}{2}$ mg and 10 mg. How much had he received total at the end of five days?

16. If LASIX® comes in a 10 ml (10 mg per ml) vial and you give $2\frac{1}{2}$ ml, how many milligrams have you given?

17. Using problem (16), how many milliliters are left in the vial?

18. The doctor orders BUMEX®(bumetanide), 2 mg daily, and you have $\frac{1}{2}$-mg tablets on hand. How many tablets would you give in a day?

19. For symptomatic relief of acute alcohol withdrawal, the doctor orders TRANXENE®, 30 mg. The tablets you have on hand are $7\frac{1}{2}$ mg. How many tablets do you give?

20. You have on hand 5-mg strength VALIUM® (diazepam) tablets. The doctor has ordered $2\frac{1}{2}$ mg t.i.d. How many tablets has the patient received at the end of the day?

Chapter 2

Decimals and Percents

This chapter is a review of decimals and percents. When you complete this chapter you should be able to:

a. Read, write, and round decimals to specific place values.
b. Add, subtract, multiply, and divide decimals.
c. Change fractions to decimals and to percents and vice-versa.
d. Use decimals and percents in working simple word problems.

2.1 Reading, Writing, and Rounding Decimals

> **PLACE VALUE - the position of a number in relation to the decimal point.**

The following table shows some of the place value names. All the names to the right of the decimal point include the letters '**th**'.

1	2	3	4	5	.	6	7	8	9	0
ten thousandths	thousands	hunderds	tens	ones		tenths	hunderdths	thousandths	ten -thousandths	hunderd-thousandths

To avoid missing the decimal point, always place a "0" in front of the decimal point when writing a decimal number less than one.

Examples: 0.65   0.01   0.125

Placing zeros after the decimal number does not change the value of the number.

Example: $0.2 = 0.20 = 0.200 = 0.2000$, etc.

TO WRITE DECIMALS USING WORD NAMES:
1. write the number to the left of the decimal point;
2. write 'and' for the decimal point;
3. write the number to the right of the decimal point;
4. write the name of the last place in the decimal number.

IF THERE IS NO NUMBER TO THE LEFT OF THE DECIMAL POINT:
1. write the number to the right of the decimal point;
2. write the name of the last place in the decimal number.

Example: Write word names for the decimal 2.5.

two	Write the number to the left of the decimal point.
and	The decimal point is represented by the word 'and'.
five	Write the number to the right of the decimal point.
tenths	Write the last place in the decimal number.

2.5 is written two and five tenths.

Example: Write word names for the decimal 0.35.

| thirty-five | Write the number to the right of the decimal point. |
| hundredths | Write the name of the last place in the decimal number. |

0.35 is written thirty-five hundredths.

Examples: Write the word names for the following decimals:

0.055   fifty-five thousandths

13.06   thirteen and six hundredths

Problems to try. Answers to these problems appear at the end of 2.1 exercises.

a.   12.025   _____

b.   0.00635   _____

Now reverse this procedure and express the following words as decimal numbers:

eight and fifteen hundredths   twenty-five thousandths

8 . 15   = 8.15   0.025

Problems to try.

c.   sixteen and twenty-four hundredths   _____

d.   one hundred sixty-five thousandths   _____

TO ROUND A NUMBER:
1. look at the digit to the right of the place to which you are rounding;
2a. if this digit is less than five, all digits to the right of the place you are rounding to become zero;
2b. if this digit is five or greater, the place you are rounding to is increased by one and every digit to the right becomes zero;
3. drop any zeros to the right of the decimal place.

Example: Round 3.47 to the nearest tenth.

3.47   4 is in the tenths place, so look at 7

3.50   7 is greater than 5, so 4 becomes 5, and 7 becomes zero

3.47 rounds to 3.5 when you drop the zero

Example: Round 7.8692 to the nearest thousandth.

7.8692   9 is in the thousandths place, so look at 2

7.8690   2 is less than 5, so 9 stays the same and 2 becomes zero

7.8692 rounds to 7.869

Example: Round 756.92 to the nearest hundred.

7̲56.92   7 is in the hundreds place, so look at 5

800.00   5 is 5 or greater, so 7 becomes 8, and 5, 6, 9, and 2 become zeros

756.92 rounds to 800

Problems to try.

e. Round 7.8692 to tenths.   _____

f. Round 124.32 to tens place.   _____

2.1   *Exercises*

Write the word names for each decimal:

1. 0.03   _____

2. 0.257   _____

3. 3.004   _____

4. 26.2   _____

5. 125.375   _____

6. 0.0035   _____

7. 6.25   _____

8. 0.0008   _____

Express the following as decimals:

9. Six and thirty-four thousandths   _____

10. Fifty-one thousandths   _____

11. One hundred sixty-five ten-thousandths   _____

12. One hundred twenty   _____

13. Forty-five and six tenths   _____

14. Nine hundred and nine hundredths   _____

15. Eighty-nine hundredths   _____

16. Thirty and five tenths   _____

Round to the nearest tenth:

17. 0.26   _____   18. 2.356   _____

19. 34.63   _____   20. 0.3334   _____

Round to the nearest hundredth:

21. 125.367   _____   22. 0.0356   _____

23. 23.6724   _____   24. 0.008   _____

Round to the nearest thousandth:

25. 56.7845   _____   26. 0.00745   _____

27. 0.7654   _____   28. 78.0836   _____

Round 6774.35279 to the nearest:

29. tenth _____   30. hundred _____

31. thousandth_____   32. hundredth _____

33. one _____   34. thousand _____

35. ten _____   36. ten-thousandths _____

Answers to Problems to try.

a. twelve and twenty-five thousandths   b. six hundred thirty-five hundred-thousandths

c. 16.24   d. 0.165   e. 7.9   f. 120

_____

Space Provided for Student Work

_____

2.2   *Adding and Subtracting Decimals*

> **TO ADD DECIMALS:**
> 1. write each number so that the decimal points are in a vertical line;
> 2. add the numbers as if there were no decimal points;
> 3. place the decimal point in the answer in line with the decimal points in the original numbers.

Example: $0.25 + 3.6 + 4 + 12.056 =$

$\begin{array}{r} 0.25 \\ 3.6 \\ 4 \\ +12.056 \\ \hline \end{array}$	Line up the decimal points.	$\begin{array}{r} 0.250 \\ 3.600 \\ 4.000 \\ +12.056 \\ \hline \end{array}$	Filling in zeros is not necessary but will help keep columns straight.

$$\begin{array}{r} 0.250 \\ 3.600 \\ 4.000 \\ +12.056 \\ \hline 19.906 \end{array}$$

Add the columns and place the decimal point in the answer in line with the other decimal points.

Example: $0.06 + 2.5 + 12.1 + 6.005 =$

$$\begin{array}{r} 0.06 \\ 2.5 \\ 12.1 \\ + \quad 6.005 \\ \hline 20.665 \end{array}$$

Problems to try. Answers to these problems appear at the end of 2.2 exercises.

a. $8.02 + 4.8 + 6 + 0.005 =$ _____

b. $0.02 + 9.009 + 11 + 0.6 =$ _____

TO SUBTRACT DECIMALS:
1. write each number so that the decimal points are in a line;
2. subtract the numbers as if there were no decimal points;
3. place the decimal point in the answer in line with the decimal points in the other numbers.

Example: $2.056 - 0.34 =$

$$\begin{array}{r} 2.056 \\ -0.34 \\ \hline \end{array}$$ Line up decimal points. $$\begin{array}{r} 2.056 \\ -0.340 \\ \hline \end{array}$$ Fill in zeros to keep columns straight.

$$\begin{array}{r} 2.056 \\ -0.340 \\ \hline 1.716 \end{array}$$ Subtract the numbers and place the decimal point in the answer in line with the other decimal points.

Example: $3.5 - 0.025 =$ $$\begin{array}{r} 3.500 \\ -0.025 \\ \hline 3.475 \end{array}$$

Problems to try.

c. $0.45 - 0.034 =$ _____

d. $12.7 - 3.245 =$ _____

2.2   Exercises

Perform the indicated operations:

1. $0.5 + 0.9$ _____   2. $7.321 + 0.53$ _____

3. $0.3 + 0.16$ _____   4. $17 + 8.34$ _____

5. 0.71 + 5.3   _____

6. 0.51 + 0.7   _____

7. 8.35 + 7.4 + 9.084   _____

8. 0.115 + 16.8 + 12 + 2.05   _____

9. 6.15 + 0.5 + 6.3 + 0.07   _____

10. 0.4 + 0.04 + 4.004   _____

11. 0.8 + 9.07 + 1908.62   _____

12. 0.746 + 9.8 + 7.22 + 393.4   _____

13. 15.4 − 8.1   _____

14. 18.2 − 18   _____

15. 2.2 − 0.35   _____

16. 69 − 35.01   _____

17. 2.07 − 0.007   _____

18. 15 − 3.9   _____

19. 20.4 − 0.4   _____

20. 16.5 − 0.0025   _____

21. 3 − 0.02   _____

22. 154.3 − 0.16   _____

23. 85.47 − 0.29   _____

24. 400.03 − 97.58   _____

25. Subtract 0.89 from 2.   _____

26. Subtract 7.3 from 18.7.   _____

27. Find the difference between 7.83 and 0.2.   _____

28. Find the difference between 41 and 8.3.   _____

29. Moe walked several times during the week. He walked 2.3 miles, 0.8 miles, 1 mile and 1.25 miles. How many miles did he walk altogether?

30. Judy started dieting and lost 9.5 lbs. the first week. The second week she gained 0.25 lbs. The third week she lost 2.75 lbs. and the fourth week she lost 1.5 lbs. How many pounds had she lost at the end of the month?

31. A baby weighed 3.69 kg at birth. At the end of one week the baby weighed 4.1 kg. How much weight did the baby gain?

32. In a 24 hour period an infant took 3.7 oz., 3.5 oz., 4 oz., and 3.25 oz. of formula. How much total formula did the infant receive?

Answers to Problems to try.

a. 18.825   b. 20.629   c. 0.416   d. 9.455

2.3   *Multiplying and Dividing Decimals*

> **TO MULTIPLY DECIMALS:**
> 1.   multiply the numbers as if there were no decimal points;
> 2.   count the number of decimal places in each number, add them together;
> 3.   put that many decimal places in the answer.

Example: $8.2 \times 0.25 =$

$$
\begin{array}{r}
8.2 \\
\times .25 \\
\hline
410 \\
164 \\
\hline
2050
\end{array} = 2.050
$$

This number contains 1 decimal place.
This number contains 2 decimal places.
All together there are 3, so the answer must have 3 decimal places.

Example: $7.8 \times 0.0003 =$

$$
\begin{array}{r}
7.8 \\
\times .0003 \\
\hline
234
\end{array} = 0.00234
$$

1 place
4 places
Add zeros to make 5 places.

Problems to try. Answers to these problems appear at the end of 2.3 exercises.

a. $10.4 \times 3.7 =$ _____

b. $0.03 \times 4.2 =$ _____

TO DIVIDE DECIMALS:
1. write the numbers in long division format;
2. if there is a decimal point in the divisor (the number you are dividing by), move it to the right until you have a whole number;
3. move the decimal point in the dividend (the number being divided) the same number of places in the same direction;
4. place the decimal point in the answer directly above the decimal point in the dividend;
5. divide as if the decimal points were not there.

Example: $9.28 \div 3.2 =$

$$3.2\overline{)9.28}$$ Move the decimal point one place to the right in the divisor and the dividend.

$$32\overline{)92.8}$$ Place the decimal point in the answer directly over the one in the dividend.

$$
\begin{array}{r}
2.9 \\
32\overline{)92.8} \\
64 \\
\hline
288 \\
288 \\
\hline
\end{array}
$$
Divide as if the decimal points were not there.

Example: $50.05 \div 0.5 =$

$$5\overline{)500.5}$$ Move the decimal points and place the decimal point in the answer.

$$
\begin{array}{r}
100.1 \\
5\overline{)500.5} \\
5 \\
\hline
005 \\
5 \\
\hline
\end{array}
$$
Divide, being careful to fill in zeros.

Example: $1 \div 4 =$

$$4 \overline{)1.00} \;\; 0.25$$

Place the decimal points, add zeros, and divide.

Zeros must be added so that division can continue

Remember: Zeros can be added after a decimal

point without changing the value.

$$\begin{array}{r} 0.25 \\ 4 \overline{)1.00} \\ \underline{8} \\ 20 \\ \underline{20} \end{array}$$

Example: $6 \div 0.25 =$

$$\begin{array}{r} 24 \\ 25 \overline{)600} \\ \underline{50} \\ 100 \\ \underline{100} \end{array}$$

Zeros had to be added to the dividend in order to move the decimal point two places.

Problems to try.

c. $0.06 \overline{)360.6}$

d. $2.5 \overline{)0.035}$

e. $8 \overline{)1}$

Sometimes the division does not come out even. When this happens, round to the nearest hundredth.

Example:

$$.666 = 0.67 \text{ or } 0.\overline{6}$$

$$3 \overline{)2} = 3 \overline{)2.000}$$

$$\begin{array}{r} \underline{18} \\ 20 \\ \underline{18} \\ 20 \\ \underline{18} \end{array}$$

The line over the 6 means that the 6 is repeating.

Example:

$$1.259 = 1.26$$

$$3.2\overline{)4.03} = 32\overline{)40.300}$$

$$\begin{array}{r} 32 \\ \hline 83 \\ 64 \\ \hline 190 \\ 160 \\ \hline 300 \\ 288 \\ \hline 12 \end{array}$$

Problems to try.

f. $6\overline{)1}$

g. $7.5\overline{)0.961}$

2.3   Exercises

Perform the indicated operations:

1. 4.002×0.03 _____

2. 5.006×0.04 _____

3. 0.0035×0.04 _____

4. 10.25×0.5 _____

5. 0.02×0.4 _____

6. 0.256×100 _____

7. 53.2×0.1 _____

8. 6.5×0.3 _____

9. 0.2×0.3 _____

10. 6.25×0.25 _____

11. 12.5×0.5 _____

12. 2.75×10.5 _____

13. $3.26 \div 0.4$ _____

14. $0.00056 \div 0.007$ _____

15. $1 \div 8$ _____

16. $12.083 \div 5.62$ _____

17. $17.5 \div 2.5$ _____

18. $31.41 \div 0.003$ _____

19. $14.7 \div 0.06$ _____

Round problems 20 to 24 to the nearest hundredth.

20. $12.1 \div 5.62$ _____

21. $1 \div 3$ _____

22. $1.566 \div 35.6$ _____

23. $15.66 \div 0.44$ _____

24. $1.174 \div 0.33$ _____

25. Multiply 0.89 times 0.32.   _____

26. Multiply 3.2 times 0.08.   _____

27. Divide 19.95 by 10.5.   _____

28.   Divide 5 into 2.   _____

29.   If the nurse gives 2.5 grains q.4h., how many grains has the patient received in
      3 days?

30.   A medication bubble pack contains 20 tablets and the doctor has ordered 1.5
      tablets t.i.d. How many whole days will the medication last?

31.   If a patient is to receive 1.5 oz. q.6h., how many whole doses does a 17 oz.
      bottle contain?

32.   If a patient receives 0.15 mg q.i.d., how many mg will the patient receive in
      5 days?

Answers to Problems to try.

a. 38.48   b. 0.126   c. 6010   d. 0.014   e. 0.125   f. 01$\overline{6}$ or 0.17   g. 0.13

Space Provided for Student Work

2.4 Converting Fractions and Decimals

TO CONVERT A FRACTION TO A DECIMAL:
1. **divide the numerator by the denominator;**
2. **round to hundredths if the division does not come out even after three places.**

Example: Convert $\frac{3}{4}$ to a decimal.

$$
\begin{array}{r}
.75 \\
4\overline{)3.00} \\
28 \\
\overline{20} \\
20 \\
\overline{}
\end{array}
$$

Divide the numerator by the denominator.

$\frac{3}{4} = 0.75$

Example: Convert $\frac{5}{6}$ to a decimal.

$$
\begin{array}{r}
.833 \\
6\overline{)5.000} \\
48 \\
\overline{20} \\
18 \\
\overline{20} \\
18 \\
\overline{2}
\end{array}
$$
repeating

$\frac{5}{6} = 0.8\overline{3}$ or 0.83

Example: Convert $\frac{27}{5}$ to a decimal.

$$
\begin{array}{r}
5.4 \\
5\overline{)27.0} \\
25 \\
\overline{20} \\
20 \\
\overline{}
\end{array}
$$

$\frac{27}{5} = 5.4$

Example: Convert $2\frac{1}{4}$ to a decimal.

Leave the whole number 2 and convert $\frac{1}{4}$ to a decimal.

$$
\begin{array}{r}
.25 \\
4\overline{\smash{)}1.00} \\
8 \\
\hline
20 \\
20 \\
\hline
\end{array}
$$

$2\frac{1}{4} = 2.25$

or

Change $2\frac{1}{4}$ to an improper fraction and divide.

$2\frac{1}{4} = \frac{9}{4}$

$$
\begin{array}{r}
2.25 \\
4\overline{\smash{)}9.00} \\
8 \\
\hline
10 \\
8 \\
\hline
20 \\
20 \\
\hline
\end{array}
$$

For any fraction with a power of 10 (10, 100, 1000, 10000, etc.) in the denominator, place the last number in the numerator in the place value defined by the denominator.

Convert $\frac{4}{10}$ to a decimal.   0.4   4 goes in the tenths place

Convert $\frac{5}{100}$ to a decimal.   0.05   5 goes in the hundredths place

Convert $\frac{24}{100}$ to a decimal.   0.24   4 goes in the hundredths place

Problems to try. Answer to these problems appear at the end of 2.4 exercises.

a.   Convert $\frac{3}{8}$ to a decimal.   _____

b.   Convert $\frac{1}{7}$ to a decimal.   _____

c.   Convert $16\frac{3}{5}$ to a decimal   _____

d.   Convert $\frac{125}{1000}$ to a decimal   _____

TO CONVERT A DECIMAL TO A FRACTION:
  1.   **the number to the left of the decimal point remains as a whole number;**
  2.   **the decimal number written without the decimal point becomes the numerator;**
  3.   **the place value of the last digit in the decimal number becomes the denominator;**
  4.   **simplify by reducing to lowest terms and/or changing to a mixed number.**

Example: Convert 0.35 to a fraction.

$\frac{35}{100}$ number without the decimal point is the numerator
5 is in the hundredths place so the denominator is 100

$\frac{35}{100} = \frac{7}{20}$ reduce to lowest terms $0.35 = \frac{7}{20}$

Example: Convert 0.005 to a fraction.

$\frac{5}{1000}$ number without the decimal point
5 is in the thousandths place

$\frac{5}{1000} = \frac{1}{200}$ reduce to lowest terms $0.005 = \frac{1}{200}$

Example: Convert 12.2 to a fraction.

Leave the whole number 12 and convert 0.2 to a fraction.

$0.2 = \frac{2}{10} = \frac{1}{5}$ so $12.2 = 12\frac{1}{5}$

or

$$\frac{122}{10} \qquad \text{number without the decimal point}$$
$$\qquad\qquad \text{last number is in the tenths place}$$

$$\frac{122}{10} = \frac{61}{5} = 12\frac{1}{5} \qquad \text{simplify by reducing and changing}$$
$$\qquad\qquad\qquad\qquad \text{to a mixed number}$$

Problems to try.

e. Convert 0.85 to a fraction.   _____

f. Convert 0.025 to a fraction   _____

g. Convert 4.5 to a fraction   _____

TO MULTIPLY A FRACTION TIMES A DECIMAL:
1. **either convert both to fractions or both to decimals;**
2. **multiply.**

Example: $\frac{1}{3} \times 2.5 =$

$$\frac{1}{3} \times \frac{25}{10} = \frac{25}{30} = \frac{5}{6} \qquad \textbf{or} \qquad 0.3 \text{ (approximately)} \times 2.5 = 0.75$$

In the example above, it is more accurate to use a fraction because of the repeating decimal. **If a fraction does not come out even as a decimal, use fractions instead of decimals to solve these kinds of problems.**

Example: $\frac{1}{2} \times 6.2 =$

$$\frac{1}{2} \times \frac{62}{10} = \frac{62}{20} = \frac{31}{10} = 3\frac{1}{10} \qquad \textbf{or} \qquad 0.5 \times 6.2 = 3.1$$

2.4   Exercises

Convert each fraction to a decimal. Round to hundredths if necessary.

1. $\frac{1}{5}$ _____

2. $\frac{7}{8}$ _____

3. $\frac{1}{40}$ _____

4. $\frac{3}{25}$ _____

5. $\frac{2}{3}$ _____

6. $\frac{3}{7}$ _____

7. $3\frac{3}{8}$ _____

8. $4\frac{1}{3}$ _____

9. $8\frac{3}{4}$ _____

10. $2\frac{5}{16}$ _____

11. $1\frac{3}{10}$ _____

12. $\frac{27}{8}$ _____

13. $21\frac{25}{100}$ _____

14. $\frac{375}{100}$ _____

15. $\frac{8}{100}$ _____

16. $\frac{35}{6}$ _____

17. $\frac{16}{10}$ _____

18. $\frac{17}{1000}$ _____

19. $\frac{13}{4}$ _____

20. $\frac{1}{1000}$ _____

Convert each decimal to a fraction. Reduce to lowest terms.

21. 0.8   _____   22. 0.65   _____

23. 0.33   _____   24. 0.006   _____

25. 0.012   _____   26. 4.4   _____

27. 2.5   _____   28. 2.05   _____

29. 0.375   _____   30. 1.004   _____

31. 8   _____   32. 12.3   _____

33. 0.36   _____   34. 20.0012   _____

35. 0.025   _____   36. 0.00125   _____

Multiply.

37. $\frac{1}{2} \times 3.5$ _____   38. $7.5 \times \frac{1}{4}$ _____

39. $12.3 \times \frac{2}{3}$ _____   40. $1\frac{1}{2} \times 0.75$ _____

Answers to Problems to try.

a. 0.375   b. 0.14   c. 16.6   d. 0.125   e. $\frac{17}{20}$ f. $\frac{1}{40}$ g. $4\frac{1}{2}$

2.5   *Converting Decimals and Percents*

TO CONVERT A DECIMAL TO A PERCENT:
1. **move the decimal point two places to the right;**
2. **add the percent sign.**

Example: Convert 0.45 to a percent.

0.45   move decimal point two places to the right

45%   add the percent sign

Example: Convert 0.006 to a percent.

0.006 = 0.6%

Example: Convert 0.2 to a percent.

0.20   add a zero so you can move two places

0.20 = 20%

Example: Convert 3 to a percent.

3.00   add two zeros

3.00 = 300%

Problems to try. Answers to these problems appear at the end of 2.5 exercises.

a. Convert 0.26 to a percent   _____

b. Convert 0.025 to a percent   _____

c. Convert 2.1 to a percent   _____

TO CONVERT A PERCENT TO A DECIMAL:
1. **drop the percent sign;**
2. **move the decimal point two places to the left.**

Example: Convert 13% to a decimal.

$$13$$ drop the percent sign

.13   move the decimal point
two places to the left   13% = 0.13

Example: Convert 12.5% to a decimal.

12.5 = 0.125

Example: Convert 6% to a decimal.

06   add a zero so you can move two places

.06 = 0.06

Example: Convert 0.3% to a decimal.

00.3   add two zeros   .003 = 0.003

Example: Convert 120% to a decimal.

120 = 1.20

Problems to try.

d. Convert 75% to a decimal.   _____

e. Convert 8% to a decimal.   _____

f. Convert 0.5% to a decimal.   _____

TO CONVERT A FRACTIONAL PERCENT TO A DECIMAL:
1.   **convert the fraction to a decimal (round to hundredths if division does not come out even); leave the percent sign (%);**
2.   **convert the percent to a decimal.**

Example: Convert $\frac{1}{2}$% to a decimal.

$\frac{1}{2} = 0.5$ convert the fraction to a decimal

$\frac{1}{2}\% = 0.5\%$ leave the percent sign

00.5 = 0.005   convert the percent to a decimal

Example: Convert $2\frac{1}{4}\%$ to a decimal.

$$2\frac{1}{4} = 2.25 \qquad\qquad \text{convert the fraction to a decimal}$$

$$2\frac{1}{4}\% = 2.25\% \qquad\qquad \text{leave the percent sign}$$

$$02.25 = 0.0225 \qquad\qquad \text{convert the percent to a decimal}$$

Example: Convert $\frac{1}{3}\%$ to a decimal.

$$\frac{1}{3} = 0.33 \qquad\qquad \text{round to hundredths}$$

$$\frac{1}{3}\% = 0.33\% \qquad\qquad \text{leave the percent sign}$$

$$00.33 = 0.0033 \qquad\qquad \text{convert the percent to a decimal}$$

Problems to try.

g. Convert $\frac{1}{8}\%$ to a decimal.   _____

h. Convert $3\frac{1}{2}\%$ to a decimal.   _____

i. Convert $6\frac{1}{9}\%$ to a decimal.   _____

2.5   *Exercises*

Convert each decimal to a percent.

1. 0.33   _____   2. 0.65   _____

3. 0.28   _____   4. 0.86   _____

5. 0.25   _____   6. 0.125   _____

7. 0.375   _____   8. 0.1275   _____

9. 0.0075   _____   10. 0.0485   _____

11. 0.3   _____   12. 0.4   _____

13. 0.8   _____   14. 1.1   _____

15. 1.5   _____   16. 0.05   _____

17. 0.03   _____   18. 2.8   _____

19. 0.5   _____   20. 0.02   _____

Convert each percent to a decimal.

21. 27%   _____   22. 85%   _____

23. 17%   _____   24. 5%   _____

25. 16%   _____   26. 3%   _____

27. 6.5%   _____   28. 1.65%   _____

29. 12.85%   _____   30. 0.3%   _____

31. 130%   _____   32. 250%   _____

33. 60%   _____   34. 9.2%   _____

35. 0.05%   _____   36. 0.01%   _____

37. 0.25%   _____   38. 2.1%   _____

39. 0.8%   _____   40. 8.9%   _____

41. $\frac{1}{8}$%   _____   42. $12\frac{1}{2}$%   _____

43. $1\frac{1}{4}$%   _____   44. $7\frac{1}{5}$%   _____

45. $\frac{2}{3}$%   _____   46. $37\frac{1}{2}$%   _____

47. $4\frac{3}{8}$%   _____   48. $2\frac{5}{6}$%   _____

49. $\frac{3}{4}$%   _____   50. $6\frac{3}{5}$%   _____

Answers to Problems to try.

a. 26%   b. 2.5%   c. 210%   d. 0.75   e. 0.08   f. 0.005   g. 0.00125   h. 0.035
i. $0.06\overline{1}$ or 0.0611

2.6   *Converting Fractions and Percents*

> **TO CONVERT A FRACTION TO A PERCENT:**
> 1. convert the fraction to a decimal;
> 2. if division does not come out even round to thousandths;
> 3. convert this decimal to a percent.

Example: Convert $\frac{3}{5}$ to a percent.

$$\frac{3}{5} = 0.6 \qquad \text{convert the fraction to a decimal}$$

$$0.60 = 60\% \qquad \text{convert the decimal to a percent}$$

Example: Convert $2\frac{1}{2}$ to a percent.

$$2\frac{1}{2} = 2.5 \qquad \text{convert the fraction to a decimal}$$

$$2.50 = 250\% \qquad \text{convert the decimal to a percent}$$

Example: Convert $\frac{7}{8}$ to a percent.

$$\frac{7}{8} = 0.875 \qquad \text{convert the fraction to a decimal}$$

$$0.875 = 87.5\% \qquad \text{convert the decimal to a percent}$$

Example: Convert $\frac{1}{3}$ to a percent.

$$\frac{1}{3} = 0.33\overline{3} \qquad \text{convert the fraction to a decimal}$$

$$0.33\overline{3} = 0.333 \qquad \text{and round to thousandths}$$

$$0.333 = 33.3\% \qquad \text{convert the decimal to a percent}$$

Problems to try. Answers to these problems appear at the end of 2.6 exercises.

a. Convert $\frac{3}{4}$ to a percent.   _____

b. Convert $\frac{5}{6}$ to a percent.   _____

c. Convert $\frac{5}{8}$ to a percent.   _____

TO CONVERT A PERCENT TO A FRACTION:
1. **convert the percent to a decimal;**
2. **convert the decimal to a fraction;**
3. **reduce the fraction to lowest terms.**

Example: Convert 65% to a fraction.

$$65\% = 0.65 \qquad \text{convert the percent to a decimal}$$

$$0.65 = \frac{65}{100} \qquad \text{convert the decimal to a fraction}$$

$$\frac{65}{100} = \frac{13}{20} \qquad \text{reduce to lowest terms}$$

Example: Convert 8% to a fraction.

$$8\% = 0.08 \qquad \text{convert the percent to a decimal}$$

$$0.08 = \frac{8}{100} \qquad \text{convert the decimal to a fraction}$$

$$\frac{8}{100} = \frac{2}{25} \qquad \text{reduce to lowest terms}$$

Example: Convert 6.5% to a fraction.

$$6.5\% = 0.065 \qquad \text{convert the percent to a decimal}$$

$$0.065 = \frac{65}{100} \qquad \text{convert the decimal to a fraction}$$

$$\frac{65}{1000} = \frac{13}{200} \qquad \text{reduce to lowest terms}$$

Problems to try.

d. Convert 36% to a fraction. _____

e. Convert 5% to a fraction. _____

f. Convert 0.25% to a fraction. _____

TO CONVERT A FRACTIONAL PERCENT TO A FRACTION:
1. **take the percent times $\frac{1}{100}$;**
2. **reduce to lowest terms.**

Example: Convert $2\frac{1}{4}\%$ to a fraction.

$$2\frac{1}{4} \times \frac{1}{100} = \frac{9}{4} \times \frac{1}{100} = \frac{9}{400} \qquad \text{reduced to lowest terms}$$

Example: Convert $12\frac{1}{2}\%$ to a fraction.

$$12\frac{1}{2} \times \frac{1}{100} = \frac{25}{2} \times \frac{1}{100} = \frac{25}{200} = \frac{1}{8} \qquad \text{reduced to lowest terms}$$

Problems to try.

g. Convert $\frac{2}{3}\%$ to a fraction. _____

h. Convert $8\frac{2}{5}\%$ to a fraction. _____

TO DETERMINE THE PERCENT STRENGTH:
1. **find the fractional part of the solution that is medication;**
2. **change this fraction to a percent.**

Example: A 400 ml solution contains 10 g of medication. What percent strength is this solution?

$$\frac{\text{medication}}{\text{solution}} = \frac{10}{400} \qquad \text{fractional part of the solution that is medication}$$

$$400 \overline{\smash{\big)}\,10.000} \;\; \underset{\text{.025}}{} = 0.025 = 2.5\% \qquad \text{change fraction to a percent}$$

$$\begin{array}{r} .025 \\ 400 \overline{\smash{\big)}\,10.000} \\ \underline{800} \\ 2000 \\ \underline{2000} \end{array}$$

Example: If you add 90 ml of sterile water to 10 ml of medication, what percent strength will you have?

10 ml medication + 90 ml sterile water = 100 ml solution

$$\frac{\text{medication}}{\text{solution}} = \frac{10}{100} \quad \text{fractional part of the solution that is medication}$$

$$\begin{array}{r} .10 \\ 100 \overline{\smash{\big)}\,10.00} \\ \underline{100} \\ 00 \end{array} = 0.10 = 10\% \qquad \text{change fraction to a percent}$$

Most common conversions.

Fraction	Decimal	Percent	Fraction	Decimal	Percent
$\frac{1}{8}$	0.125	12.5%	$\frac{1}{6}$	0.166	16.6%
$\frac{1}{4}$	0.25	25%	$\frac{1}{3}$	0.333	33.3%
$\frac{3}{8}$	0.375	37.5%	$\frac{2}{3}$	0.667	66.7%
$\frac{1}{2}$	0.5	50%	$\frac{5}{6}$	0.833	83.3%
$\frac{5}{8}$	0.625	62.5%	$\frac{1}{20}$	0.05	5%
$\frac{3}{4}$	0.75	75%	$\frac{1}{100}$	0.01	1%
$\frac{7}{8}$	0.875	87.5%	$\frac{1}{200}$	0.005	0.5% or $\frac{1}{2}$%

2.6 Exercises

Convert each fraction to a percent.

1. $\frac{1}{40}$ _____   2. $\frac{11}{15}$ _____

3. $2\frac{2}{5}$ _____   4. $\frac{4}{5}$ _____

5. $\frac{1}{50}$ _____   6. $\frac{9}{8}$ _____

7. $\frac{2}{7}$ _____   8. $\frac{3}{8}$ _____

9. $\frac{3}{20}$ _____   10. $\frac{1}{400}$ _____

11. $\frac{1}{4}$ _____   12. $\frac{3}{16}$ _____

13. $\frac{2}{3}$ _____   14. $\frac{5}{100}$ _____

15. $\frac{1}{1000}$ _____

Convert each percent to a fraction.

16. 25% _____   17. 300% _____

18. 15% _____   19. 20% _____

20. 8% _____

21. 80% _____

22. 0.5% _____

23. 0.005% _____

24. 0.05% _____

25. 2.5% _____

26. $\frac{3}{8}$% _____

27. $37\frac{1}{2}$% _____

28. $6\frac{1}{4}$% _____

29. $33\frac{1}{3}$% _____

30. $\frac{1}{2}$% _____

31. 7.5% _____

32. 6.25% _____

33. 4% _____

34. 150% _____

35. 0.2% _____

36. Fill in the table.

Fraction	Decimal	Percent	Fraction	Decimal	Percent
$\frac{3}{40}$				0.025	
	0.45		$\frac{1}{20}$		
		$\frac{3}{4}$%			25%
$2\frac{1}{5}$				3.2	
	0.008				0.3%

37. If a patient uses 8 oz. out of a 12 oz. bottle of medicine, what percent of the whole bottle has he used?

38. A patient has 30 tablets of medication. If he takes 24 of these, what percent are left?

39. There is 5 ml of medication in a 20 ml bottle of solution. What is the percent of medication to solution?

40. If you add 145 ml of sterile water to 5 ml of medication, what percent strength solution will you have?

Answers to Problems to try.

a. 75%   b. 83.3%   c. 62.5%   d. $\frac{9}{25}$ e. $\frac{1}{20}$ f. $\frac{1}{400}$ g. $\frac{1}{150}$ h. $\frac{21}{250}$

Space Provided for Student Work

2.7   *Word Problems*

> **REMEMBER**
>   Total medication = Amount per tablet × Number of tablets
>   Number of tablets = Total medication ÷ Amount per tablet

Read the problem to determine what information is given and what must be found.

Look for words that give a hint as to whether you should add, subtract, multiply or divide to get the answer.

When you get the answer, go back and read the problem again to see if your answer makes sense.

Example: You give a patient three tablets from a bottle labeled 0.75 grain each. How much medication has he received?

Number of tablets = 3

Amount per tablet = 0.75

Total medication = 3 × 0.75 = 2.25 grain

Example: To give 7.5 mg of medication from 15 mg tablets, how many tablets should be given?

Total medication = 7.5 mg

Amount per tablet = 15 mg

Number of tablets = 7.5 ÷ 15 = 0.5 tablet

Example: Marc started his diet weighing 189 lbs. 5 oz. The first week he lost 5 lbs. 12 oz., the second week he lost 3.25 lbs., and the third week he gained 1.5 lbs. What was his weight at the end of the third week?

The first thing you need to do in this problem is to either change to pounds and ounces or all pounds with decimals.

a. **Approach 1:**
Change to pounds and ounces, remembering that 16 oz. = 1 lb.

3.25 lbs. = 3 lbs. and 0.25 × 16 = 3 lbs. 4 oz.

1.5 lbs. = 1 lbs. and 0.5 × 16 = 1 lbs. 8 oz.

Now add and subtract to find the answer.

Total loss =	5 lbs. 12 oz.	Beginning wt.	189 lbs. 5 oz.
	+3 lbs. 4 oz.	Plus gain	+ 1 lb. 8 oz.
	8 lbs. 16 oz.		190 lbs. 13 oz.

190 lbs. 13 oz.	borrow	189 lbs. 29 oz.	
−8 lbs. 16 oz.		−8 lbs. 16 oz.	
		181 lbs. 13 oz.	Answer

b. **Approach 2:**
Change ounces to decimals.

189 lbs. 5 oz. = 189 lbs. + $\frac{5}{16}$ = 189 + 0.3125 = 189.3125 lbs.

5 lbs. 12 oz. = 5 lbs. + $\frac{12}{16}$ = 5 + 0.75 = 5.75 lbs.

Total loss =	5.75 lbs.	Beginning wt.	189.3125 lbs.
	+3.25 lbs.	Plus gain	+1.5 lbs.
	9 lbs.		190.8125 lbs.

190.8125
−9
———
181.8125 lbs. = 181 lbs. + (0.8125 × 16 oz.) = 181 lbs. 13 oz.

2.7   *Exercises*

1. If you give one tablet daily of PREMARIN® 0.625 mg for 5 days, how many milligrams total have you given?

2. If a subcutaneous pain pump is set to deliver 15.5 mg of DILAUDID® every hour, how much medication has the patient received after $7\frac{1}{2}$ hours?

3. 5 ml of medication are added to 795 ml of sterile water. What is the solution strength expressed as a percent?

4. If a patient receives $\frac{1}{4}$ of a 1-grain morphine sulfate tablet, what percent of the tablet did the patient receive?

5. LANOXIN® pediatric elixir comes in a 60 ml bottle. There are 0.05 mg of medication in every ml. How many total milligrams are contained in the bottle?

6. If a patient takes 0.6 mg nitroglycerin sublingually every 5 minutes for 3 doses, what is the total medication received?

7. A 3-year-old with pneumonia is given cefotaxime, 325 mg q.6h. You have on hand a solution that contains 50 mg of cefotaxime in every milliliter of solution. How many milliliters will you give?

8. Carol's time breakdown for one day showed her hours worked as follows: office, 2.5 hr.; travel, 1.75 hr.; field, 3.25 hr. What were her total hours for the day?

9. Dave started his diet weighing 179.5 lbs. The first week he lost 5.75 lbs., the second week he lost 3.25 lbs., the third week he gained 1.5 lbs., and the fourth week he lost 1.75 lbs. What was his weight at the end of the fourth week? How many pounds had he lost?

10. The following doses of a medication are given during the week: 1.5 mg, 2.5 mg, 1.25 mg, 3 mg, 4.25 mg. What is the total dose given?

11. Using problem 10, how much more medication is needed to total 15 mg?

12. If the doctor ordered a total of 17.5 mg of medication to be equally divided over a period of 7 days, how much would you give each day?

13. Kurt ran 4.2 miles on Monday, 7.7 miles on Tuesday, and 8.4 miles on Wednesday. How many miles did he run in the 3 days?

14. In problem 13, how many more miles would he have to run to reach his goal of 50 miles per week?

15. A newborn weighed 7 lbs. 6 oz. before being taken out to breast feed. When he returned, his weight was 7 lbs. 8.5 oz. How much did he gain?

16. Margaret's total hours for the week were as follows: Monday, 7.5 hrs.; Tuesday, 8 hrs.; Wednesday, 9.75 hrs.; Thursday, 8.25 hrs.; and Friday, 7.75 hrs. What are her total hours for the week?

17. If Margaret is supposed to work a 40-hour week, how many hours of overtime did she have in problem 16?

18. Peggy worked 37.5 hours each week. She has a five-day work week. On the average, how many hours per day does she work?

19. A patient was weighed weekly and showed the following losses: first week, 2.25 lbs.; second week, 1.5 lbs.; third week, 0.75 lbs.; fourth week, 3.5 lbs. What was the total weight loss for the four weeks?

20. If you give 25 mg of VALIUM® (diazepam) each day for 14 days, what is the total dosage received?

21. If you give 1.5 mg of medication q.i.d., what is the total dosage for 1 week?

22. The patient received a total of 70 mg of medication in one week in divided doses q.i.d. Each dose contained how many mg?

23. If Carol lost 15 lbs. in 4 weeks, what is her average weekly weight loss?

24. A patient takes 7 tablets out of a bottle containing 28 tablets. What percent of the total tablets available has she received?

25. You have a bottle labeled 1 gram of medication in 200 ml of solution. What is the percent strength?

26. Kelly started out his diet weighing 225.75 lbs. The first week he lost 10 lbs. 6 oz., the second week he lost 9 lbs. 4 oz., the third week he gained 0.75 lbs., and the fourth week he lost 7.5 lbs. What was his weight at the end of the fourth week? What was his total weight loss?

27. The doctor ordered 0.50 g of medication. You have 0.25 g tablets. How many tablets will you give?

Chapter 2 Test

Round 1255.6253 to the nearest:

1. tenth _____   2. hundred _____

3. thousandth _____   4. hundredth _____

Perform the indicated operations. Round to hundredths when necessary.

5. $60.05 + 0.125$ _____   6. $8 - 0.75$ _____

7. 0.4×1.2 _____   8. $0.4 \div 1.2$ _____

9. $10.34 - 7$ _____   10. 0.0025×16 _____

11. $3 \div 16$ _____   12. $1.18 \div 0.3$ _____

13. $6.57 + 8.102 + 2$ _____   14. 2.5×10.75 _____

15. $3.05 - 0.005$ _____   16. $0.3 + 0.003 + 3$ _____

17. $3\frac{1}{4} \times 0.8$ _____   18. $0.05 \times 7\frac{1}{2}$ _____

19. $\frac{1}{6} \times 4.5$ _____

20. Fill in the table.

Fraction	Decimal	Percent	Fraction	Decimal	Percent
$\frac{7}{40}$				0.0005	
	0.85		$\frac{7}{500}$		
$1\frac{1}{5}$					0.01%
		3%			$1\frac{3}{5}\%$

21. Joe walked 3.6 miles, 0.9 miles, 2 miles, 2.25 miles and 1.3 miles in one week. How many total miles did he walk?

22. In problem 21, was Joe over or under his goal of 12 miles per week? By how much?

23. A newborn weighed 6 lbs. 8 oz. The first day she lost 2.5 oz., the second day she gained 0.75 oz., and the third day she gained 0.85 oz. What did she weigh when she went home on the fourth day?

24. A patient receives 1.25 mg of medication t.i.d. How much total medication has the patient received in 5 days?

25. Marc takes 3 tablets each containing 0.15 mg of medication. How much total medication has Marc taken?

26. The doctor orders 15 mg daily to be divided into 6 doses. How much is in each dose?

27. You have tablets containing 12.5 mg each. The patient must receive a total of 37.5 mg. How many tablets will the patient receive?

28. The doctor orders 4 ml q.6h. for 6 days. You have a bottle containing 75 ml. How many whole doses can you get out of the bottle? Will this bottle last for 6 days?

29. A patient has been taking 0.25 g of a medication daily. If she has taken a total of 1.75 g, how many days has she been taking the medication?

30. You have a bottle labeled 5 mg of medication in 200 ml of solution. What is the percent strength?

Chapter 3

Ratios and Proportions

This chapter is a review of ratios and proportions. When you complete this chapter you should be able to:

a. Reduce and simplify ratios.
b. Identify and solve proportions.
c. Change ratio strength to percent strength and vice versa.
d. Solve word problems using proportions.

3.1 Ratios

> **RATIO** is a fraction that shows the relationship of one whole number to another.

Ratios will usually be written in one of three ways. The ratio of A to B may be written: A to B   A:B $\frac{A}{B}$

Example: Write the ratio of 12 to 5.

$$12 \text{ to } 5 \qquad 12:5 \qquad \frac{12}{5}$$

> **TO SIMPLIFY A RATIO:**
> 1. convert both quantities to the same units if necessary;
> 2. convert both quantities from decimals to whole numbers if necessary;
> 3. reduce this result to lowest terms as you would a fraction.

Example: Simplify the ratio 48 to 30.

$$\frac{48}{30} = \frac{8}{5} \quad \textbf{or} \quad 8{:}5 \quad \textbf{or} \quad 8 \text{ to } 5$$

Example: Simplify the ratio 42:156.

$$\frac{42}{156} = \frac{7}{26} \quad \textbf{or} \quad 7{:}26 \quad \textbf{or} \quad 7 \text{ to } 26$$

Example: Simplify the ratio 20 minutes to 1 hour.

First convert 1 hour to 60 minutes, then reduce the resulting fraction.

$$\frac{20 \text{ min.}}{60 \text{ min.}} = \frac{1}{3} \quad \textbf{or} \quad 1{:}3 \quad \textbf{or} \quad 1 \text{ to } 3$$

Example: Simplify the ratio 3 gallons to 3 quarts (4 qt. = 1 gal.).

$$\frac{3 \text{ gal.}}{3 \text{ qt.}} = \frac{12 \text{ qt.}}{3 \text{ qt.}} = \frac{4}{1} \quad \textbf{or} \quad 4{:}1 \quad \textbf{or} \quad 4 \text{ to } 1$$

Example: Simplify the ratio 0.3 grams to 0.5 grams.

$$\frac{0.3 \text{ g}}{0.5 \text{ g}}$$ Move the decimal point one place to the right in both the numerator and the denominator. $= \dfrac{3}{5}$

This is the same as multiplying both the numerator and denominator by 10.

Example: Simplify the ratio 0.05 grams to 0.2 grams.

$$\frac{0.05 \text{ g}}{0.2 \text{ g}}$$ Move the decimal point two places to the right in both the numerator and the denominator and reduce.

$$\frac{5}{20} = \frac{1}{4}$$

This is the same as multiplying the numerator and the denominator by 100.

Example: Simplify the ratio $2\frac{1}{2}$ cups to $3\frac{1}{3}$ cups.

Simplify as you would a complex fraction.

$$\frac{2\frac{1}{2}}{3\frac{1}{2}} = 2\frac{1}{2} \div 3\frac{1}{3} = \frac{5}{2} \times \frac{3}{10} = \frac{15}{20} = \frac{3}{4}$$

Problems to try. Answers to these problems appear at the end of 3.1 exercises.

Simplify these ratios.

a. 125 mg to 375 mg   _____

b. 16 hr. to 3 days   _____

c. 0.25 liters to 1.5 liters   _____

d. $\frac{1}{3}$ gal. to $1\frac{1}{2}$ gal.   _____

RATE   is a ratio of two numbers having different units of measure that cannot be converted to the same units.

TO SIMPLIFY A RATE:
1.   **reduce as is and leave the unit names in the answer;**
2.   **rates can be expressed as decimal numbers or fractions.**

Example: Simplify the ratio 6 quarts to 2 pounds.

Since pounds and quarts cannot be changed to the same unit, reduce the fraction $\frac{6}{2}$ to $\frac{3}{1}$ and write:

3 qt. to 1 lb.   **or** $\frac{3 \text{ qt.}}{1 \text{ lb.}}$ **or**   3 qt. per lb.   **or**   3 qt./lb.

If you want to express the rate per one unit, divide the numerator by the denominator.

Example: A pipe can fill a 125-gallon tank with water in 2 hours. What is the rate in gallons per hour?

$$\frac{\text{gal.}}{\text{hr.}} = \frac{125}{2} = 125 \div 2 = 62.5 \text{ gal. per hr.}$$

Example: A patient receives 1000 ml IV solution in 12 hours. What is the rate in ml per hour? (round to tenths)

$$\frac{\text{ml}}{\text{hr.}} = \frac{1000}{12} = 1000 \div 12 = 83.3 \text{ ml/hr.}$$

Problems to try.

Simplify these rates.

e. 1500 ml to 24 hr. _____

f. 45 gal. to 3 hr. _____

3.1 Exercises

Simplify these ratios (round to tenths when necessary).

1. 5 nickels to $2 _____

2. 60 mg to 390 mg _____

3. 8 hours to 3 days _____

4. 4 days to 2 weeks _____

5. 3 feet to 8 inches   _____

6. 6 qt. to 2 gal.   _____

7. 60 men to 80 men   _____

8. 360 grains to 80 grains   _____

9. 0.75 grams to 1.2 grams   _____

10. 2.3 kg to 46 kg   _____

11. 2.25 liters to 1.3 liters _____

12. 0.15 mg to 200 mg   _____

13. 0.8 kg to 0.5 kg   _____

14. 0.35 g to 1.05 g   _____

15. $\frac{1}{5}$ gal. to $\frac{2}{3}$ gal.   _____

16. $12\frac{1}{2}$ lb. to $9\frac{3}{8}$ lb.   _____

17. $\frac{7}{8}$ oz. to $3\frac{1}{2}$ oz.   _____

18. $2\frac{2}{3}$ drams to 3 drams   _____

19. 12 feet in 2 minutes   _____

20. 8 women to 40 men   _____

21. 500 ml in 6 hours   _____

22. 1.5 ml to 100 mg   _____

23. A patient receives 1200 ml of IV solution in 12 hours. What is the rate in ml per hour?

24. Out of a total of 56 patients, 32 are men. What is the ratio of women to men?

25. The label on a medication reads 5 mg = 10 ml. How many mg are there per milliliter?

26. The label on a medication has a ratio strength of $\frac{150 \text{ mg}}{100 \text{ ml}}$. What is the strength per ml?

27. A patient receives 500 ml of IV fluid in 12 hours. What is the rate in ml per hour?

28. A patient receives 1000 ml of IV fluid in 8 hours. What is the rate in ml per hour?

29. The label on a medication reads 250 mg/20 ml. How may mg are there per milliliter?

30. There are 36 women and 15 men patients. What is the ratio of men to the total number of patients?

Answers to Problems to try.

a. $\dfrac{1}{3}$ b. $\dfrac{2}{9}$ c. $\dfrac{1}{6}$ d. $\dfrac{2}{9}$ e. 62.5 ml/hr. or $\dfrac{125 \text{ ml}}{2 \text{ hr.}}$ f. 15 gal. per hr.

Space Provided for Student Work

3.2 Proportions

PROPORTION is a statement that two ratios are equal. $\dfrac{a}{b} = \dfrac{c}{d}$

---

a and d are called the extremes
b and c are called the means

A proportion is true only if the product of the extremes equals the product of the means, in other words if **a** times **d** (ad) equals **b** times **c** (bc). This is also referred to as cross products. **ad = bc**

Example: Do the ratios $\dfrac{16}{6}$ and $\dfrac{8}{3}$ form a proportion?

Does $16 \times 3 = 6 \times 8$? $48 = 48$

So $\dfrac{16}{6} = \dfrac{8}{3}$ and these ratios form a proportion.

Example: Do the ratios $\dfrac{5}{12}$ and $\dfrac{3}{7}$ form a proportion?

Does $5 \times 7 = 12 \times 3$? $35 \neq 36$

(the symbol $\neq$ means "not equal to.")

So $\dfrac{5}{12} \neq \dfrac{3}{7}$ and these ratios do not form a proportion.

Example: Do the ratios $\dfrac{\frac{1}{2}}{1\frac{1}{3}} = \dfrac{3}{5}$ form a proportion?

Does $\dfrac{1}{2} \times 5 = 1\dfrac{1}{3} \times 3$? $\dfrac{1}{2} \times \dfrac{5}{1} = \dfrac{5}{2} = 2\dfrac{1}{2}$

$\dfrac{4}{3} \times \dfrac{3}{1} = \dfrac{12}{3} = 4$

$2\dfrac{1}{2} \neq 4$ So these ratios do not form a proportion.

Problems to try. Answers to these problems appear at the end of 3.2 exercises.

Do these ratios form proportions?

a. $\dfrac{15}{6}, \dfrac{45}{18}$ _____

b. $\dfrac{6}{31}, \dfrac{5}{26}$ _____

c. $\dfrac{\frac{1}{3}}{\frac{1}{2}}, \dfrac{30}{45}$ _____

d. $\dfrac{1.7}{18}, \dfrac{0.68}{7.2}$ _____

When three of the four terms of a proportion are known, it is possible to find the value of the unknown term.

TO SOLVE A PROPORTION:
1. set the product of the extremes equal to the product of the means (set the cross products equal);
2. divide each product by the number by which the unknown term is multiplied (the number preceding the X).

Example: $\dfrac{2}{3} = \dfrac{X}{51}$ $51(2) = 3X$ set cross products equal

$102 = 3X$ do the multiplication

$\dfrac{102}{3} = \dfrac{3X}{3}$ divide by the number preceding the X

$34 = X$

Example: $\dfrac{X}{8} = \dfrac{2\frac{1}{4}}{18}$ $18X = 8(2\frac{1}{4})$ set cross products equal

$18X = \dfrac{8}{1} \cdot \dfrac{9}{4}$

$18X = 18$ do the multiplication

$\dfrac{18X}{18} = \dfrac{18}{18}$ divide by the number preceding the X

$X = 1$

Example: $\dfrac{2.7}{0.45} = \dfrac{X}{5}$ $2.7(5) = 0.45X$ set cross products equal

$13.5 = 0.45X$ do the multiplication

$\dfrac{13.5}{0.45} = \dfrac{0.45X}{0.45}$ divide by the number preceding X

$30 = X$

Problems to try.

e. $\dfrac{3}{X} = \dfrac{21}{14}$ _____

f. $\dfrac{X}{\frac{1}{2}} = \dfrac{10}{15}$ _____

g. $\dfrac{3.2}{4.8} = \dfrac{4}{X}$ _____

3.2 Exercises

Do these ratios form proportions?

1. $\dfrac{\frac{1}{2}}{2\frac{1}{2}}, \dfrac{3}{10}$ _____   2. $\dfrac{16}{13}, \dfrac{15}{12}$ _____

3. $\dfrac{\frac{2}{3}}{2\frac{1}{2}}, \dfrac{8}{30}$ _____   4. $\dfrac{2\frac{1}{2}}{3\frac{1}{4}}, \dfrac{20}{25}$ _____

5. $\dfrac{\frac{1}{3}}{\frac{1}{4}}, \dfrac{\frac{1}{2}}{\frac{3}{8}}$ _____   6. $\dfrac{1.3}{24}, \dfrac{0.52}{0.96}$ _____

7. $\dfrac{126}{750}, \dfrac{84}{500}$ _____   8. $\dfrac{1.75}{2.5}, \dfrac{20}{49}$ _____

9. $\dfrac{3.2}{7.2}, \dfrac{0.4}{0.9}$ _____

10. $\dfrac{0.2}{0.5}, \dfrac{\frac{1}{6}}{\frac{5}{12}}$ _____

Solve these proportions.

11. $\dfrac{2}{X} = \dfrac{8}{10}$ _____

12. $\dfrac{5}{8} = \dfrac{X}{48}$ _____

13. $\dfrac{2}{7} = \dfrac{36}{X}$ _____

14. $\dfrac{\frac{2}{3}}{X} = \dfrac{9}{27}$ _____

15. $\dfrac{X}{18} = \dfrac{\frac{2}{3}}{6}$ _____

16. $\dfrac{0.8}{5} = \dfrac{X}{10}$ _____

17. $\dfrac{\frac{1}{3}}{\frac{1}{4}} = \dfrac{X}{4}$ _____

18. $\dfrac{0.2}{70} = \dfrac{X}{100}$ _____

19. $\dfrac{0.4}{0.5} = \dfrac{X}{10}$ _____

20. $\dfrac{0.25}{0.5} = \dfrac{8}{X}$ _____

21. $\dfrac{\frac{2}{3}}{\frac{1}{5}} = \dfrac{25}{X}$ _____

22. $\dfrac{0.36}{0.27} = \dfrac{X}{3}$ _____

23. $\dfrac{2\frac{1}{2}}{7\frac{1}{2}} = \dfrac{X}{5}$ _____

24. $\dfrac{X}{3} = \dfrac{7.5}{9}$ _____

25. $\dfrac{0.039}{0.06} = \dfrac{0.13}{X}$ _____

26. $\dfrac{125}{750} = \dfrac{X}{500}$ _____

27. $\dfrac{0.15}{500} = \dfrac{X}{1000}$ _____   28. $\dfrac{5}{100} = \dfrac{0.2}{X}$ _____

29. $\dfrac{200}{5} = \dfrac{120}{X}$ _____   30. $\dfrac{50}{1000} = \dfrac{2.5}{X}$ _____

Answers to Problems to try.

a. yes   b. no   c. yes   d. yes   e. 2   f. $\dfrac{1}{3}$ g. 6

Space Provided for Student Work

3.3   Converting Ratio Strength and Percent Strength

> **RATIO STRENGTH   is a fraction comparing the amount of medication by weight in a solution to the total amount of solution.**

Example: What is the ratio strength of a 50 ml solution containing 3 grams of medication?

$$\frac{3 \text{ grams}}{50 \text{ ml}} \quad \textbf{or} \quad 3 \text{ g:}50 \text{ ml} \quad \textbf{or} \quad 3 \text{ g} = 50 \text{ ml} \quad \textbf{or} \quad 3 \text{ g to } 50 \text{ ml}$$

> **PERCENT STRENGTH   represents the amount of grams of medication in 100 ml of solution.**

Example: What does 6% strength mean?

$$\frac{6 \text{ grams}}{100 \text{ ml}} \quad \textbf{or} \quad 6 \text{ g:}100 \text{ ml} \quad \textbf{or} \quad 6 \text{ g} = 100 \text{ ml} \quad \textbf{or} \quad 6 \text{ g to } 100 \text{ ml}$$

In the two examples above, does the ratio strength equal the percent strength? Use the rule for proportions to see that they do.

$$\frac{3}{50} = \frac{6}{100} \qquad 3(100) = 50(6) \quad 300 = 300$$

We can use this principle to convert ratio strength to percent strength.

> **TO CONVERT FROM RATIO STRENGTH TO PERCENT STRENGTH:**
> 1. the ratio strength will be one side of the proportion;
> 2. the percent strength ($\frac{X}{100}$) will be the other side of the proportion;
> 3. solve the proportion;
> 4. place a percent sign after the solution.
>
> **or**
>
> Use the rule for converting a fraction to a percent.

Example: Convert $\frac{5 \text{ g}}{20 \text{ ml}}$ to percent strength.

$$\frac{5}{20} = \frac{X}{100} \qquad \text{set up the proportion}$$

$$5(100) = 20 X$$

$$500 = 20 X$$

$$\frac{500}{20} = X = 25 \quad \text{solve the proportion}$$

$$\frac{5 \text{ g}}{20 \text{ ml}} = 25\% \quad \text{add the percent sign}$$

Example: 500 ml of solution contain 25 grams of medication. What is the percent strength?

$$\frac{25 \text{ g}}{500 \text{ ml}} = \frac{X}{100} \qquad \text{set up the proportion}$$

$$25(100) = 500 X$$

$$2500 = 500 X$$

$$\frac{2500}{500} = X = 5 \qquad \text{solve the proportion}$$

$$\frac{25 \text{ g}}{500 \text{ ml}} = 5\% \qquad \text{add the percent sign}$$

Example: What percent strength is the ratio 1:400?

$$\frac{1 \text{ g}}{400 \text{ ml}} = \frac{X}{100} \qquad \text{set up the proportion}$$

$$100 = 400 X$$

$$\frac{100}{400} = X = 0.25 \quad \text{solve the proportion}$$

$$1:400 = 0.25\% \quad \text{add the percent sign}$$

Problems to try. Answers to these problems appear at the end of 3.3 exercises.

Change to percent strength.

a. 2 g = 20 ml   _____

b. 1:1000   _____

c. $\dfrac{3\,g}{25\,ml}$ _____

TO CONVERT FROM PERCENT STRENGTH TO RATIO STRENGTH:
1. place the percent strength, without the percent sign, over 100;
2. if necessary convert this fraction to the form of one whole number to another (no decimals or fractions);
3. reduce this fraction to lowest terms.

or

Use the rule for converting a percent to a fraction.

Example: Convert 8% to ratio strength.

$\dfrac{8}{100} = \dfrac{2}{25} = \dfrac{2\,g}{25\,ml}$ place percent strength over 100 and reduce

Example: Convert 0.5% to ratio strength.

$\dfrac{0.5}{100}$ place the percent strength over 100

        eliminate the decimal point by moving it one place

$\dfrac{5}{1000}$ to the right in both numerator and denominator

$\dfrac{5}{1000} = \dfrac{1}{200}$ or 1:200   then reduce

Example: Convert $2\frac{1}{2}\%$ to ratio strength.

$$\frac{2\frac{1}{2}}{100} \qquad \text{place the percent strength over 100}$$

$$\frac{5}{2} \div \frac{100}{1} = \frac{5}{2} \times \frac{1}{100} = \frac{5}{200} = \frac{1}{40} \quad \text{simplify and reduce}$$

Problems to try.

Convert to ratio strength.

d. 1% _____

e. 0.01% _____

f. $1\frac{1}{3}\%$ _____

Ratios are the preferred way to write extremely small concentrations. For example, a concentration of 0.01% would probably be written 1:10000.

3.3 Exercises

1. What does 8% strength mean? _____

2. What does 24% strength mean? _____

3. What does $7\frac{1}{2}\%$ strength mean? _____

4. What does the ratio strength $\frac{8}{50}$ mean? _____

5.   What does the ratio strength 1:100 mean?   _____

6.   What does the ratio strength 15 to 200 mean?   _____

Convert to percent strength (round to tenths when necessary).

7.   1:40   _____   8.   3:4   _____

9.   1:15   _____   10.   1:10000   _____

11.   1:250   _____   12.   2:200   _____

13.   3 g:150 ml   _____   14.   1 g/4000 ml   _____

15.   10 g = 500 ml   _____   16.   1:1500   _____

17.   1:2000   _____   18.   5 g to 2500 ml   _____

Convert to ratio strength.

19.   10%   _____   20.   7.5%   _____

21. $5\frac{1}{4}\%$ _____   22. $1\frac{1}{2}\%$ _____

23.   0.25%   _____   24.   0.001%   _____

25. 0.04%   _____   26. 2.5%   _____

27. $12\frac{1}{2}\%$ _____   28. $\frac{1}{3}\%$ _____

29. $\frac{1}{2}\%$ _____   30. 0.05%   _____

Answers to Problems to try.

a. 10%   b. 0.1%   c. 12%   d. 1:100   e. 1:10000   f. 1:75

Space Provided for Student Work

3.4   Word Problems

Proportions can be used to solve many word problems.

TO SOLVE A WORD PROBLEM USING PROPORTIONS:
1. place the given ratio, with units, on one side of the proportion;
2. on the other side of the proportion, write the corresponding units from this ratio (so that the corresponding units are the same);
3. place the third number in the problem with the correct unit in the second ratio;
4. place an X in the other part of this ratio;
5. solve the proportion;
6. label the answer.

Example: In 4 days, Jane ran 50 miles. At this rate, how long would it take her to run 120 miles?

$$\frac{4 \text{ days}}{50 \text{ miles}} = \frac{\text{days}}{\text{miles}}$$ the given ratio on one side with the

corresponding units on the other

$$\frac{4 \text{ days}}{50 \text{ miles}} = \frac{\text{X days}}{120 \text{ miles}}$$ 120 goes with miles and X with days

$4(120) = 50 \text{ X}$

$480 = 50 \text{ X}$

$480 \div 50 = \text{X} = 9.6$ solve the proportion

9.6 days or about 10 days   label your answer

Example: Joan drinks 2 pints of milk in 3 days. At this rate, how many pints will she drink in one week?

$$\frac{2 \text{ pints}}{3 \text{ days}} = \frac{\text{pints}}{\text{days}}$$ ratio on one side with units on the other

$$\frac{2 \text{ pints}}{3 \text{ days}} = \frac{\text{X pints}}{7 \text{ days}}$$ 7 goes with the days and X with the pints

or   This proportion could also be written as follows: (The key is to have the same units on the top and the same units on the bottom.

$$\frac{3 \text{ days}}{2 \text{ pints}} = \frac{7 \text{ days}}{X \text{ pints}}$$

$3 X = 2(7)$

$3 X = 14$

$14 \div 3 = X = 4\frac{2}{3}$ or 4.7   solve the proportion

$4\frac{2}{3}$ pints   label your answer

Example: How many grams of medication are in 300 ml of an 8% solution?

8% means $\frac{8 \text{ grams}}{100 \text{ ml}}$

$\frac{8 \text{ grams}}{100 \text{ ml}} = \frac{\text{grams}}{\text{ml}}$ ratio and units

$\frac{8 \text{ grams}}{100 \text{ ml}} = \frac{X \text{ grams}}{300 \text{ ml}}$ 300 with the ml and X with the grams

$8(300) = 100 X$

$2400 = 100 X$

$2400 \div 100 = X = 24 \text{ grams}$ solve the proportion and label

Example: You are to give a patient 75 mg of medication. You have 25 mg tablets available. How may tablets will you give the patient?

$\frac{25 \text{ mg}}{1 \text{ tab}} = \frac{75 \text{ mg}}{X \text{ tab}}$ set up proportion

$1(75) = 25 X$

$75 \div 25 = 3 \text{ tablets}$ solve the proportion and label

3.4   Exercises

Solve using proportions.

1. If a 15% solution contains 45 grams of medication, how many ml of solution do you have?

2. A certain medication is given according to body weight. Dosage is $\frac{1}{2}$ teaspoon for every 15 pounds of body weight. How many teaspoons do you give a woman weighing 120 pounds?

3. A patient is to receive 500 mg of medication per day. The medication is available in 125 mg tablets. How many tablets should you give?

4. You are to give a patient $3\frac{3}{4}$ grains of medication from $1\frac{1}{2}$ grain tablets. How many tablets should you give?

5. The label on a medication reads: 10 mg per kilogram of body weight. How many mg would you give a patient weighing 47 kilograms?

6. The label on a medication reads: 20 mg per 5 kg of body weight. How many mg would you give a patient weighing 52 kg?

7. The label on a medication reads: 300 mg per tablet. If you are to give the patient $2\frac{1}{2}$ tablets, how many mg of medication will the patient receive?

8. The strength available is 25 mg in 1.5 ml. A dosage of 15 mg has been ordered. How many ml do you give the patient?

9. You have available a dosage strength of 6 mg to 2 ml. How many ml do you give a patient who needs 4 mg?

10. The strength available is 100 mg = 1.5 ml. A dosage of 250 mg has been ordered. How many ml do you give the patient?

11. Jason uses three 8 oz. bottles of MAALOX® in two weeks. At this rate, how many ounces will he take in 3 weeks? How many 8 oz. bottles will he need for a 3-week supply?

12. How many grams of medication are in 250 ml of a $7\frac{1}{2}$% solution?

13. The label on a medication reads: 25 mg per kilogram of body weight per day. How much would you give a patient weighing 68 kg? If he were given the medication four times a day, how many mg would he take in each dose?

14. The strength available is 250 mg = 5 ml. A dosage of 75 mg has been ordered. How many ml do you give the patient?

15. You are to give a patient $3\frac{3}{4}$ grains of medication from $2\frac{1}{2}$-grain tablets. How many tablets do you give?

Chapter 3 Test

Simplify these ratios.

1. 2 days to 15 hours   _____

2. 0.8 g to 1.2 g   _____

3. $6\frac{1}{2}$ lb. to $8\frac{2}{3}$ lb.   _____

4. The label on a medication reads 350 mg per 10 ml. How many mg are there per milliliter?

        _____

Solve these proportions.

5. $\dfrac{\frac{5}{8}}{2} = \dfrac{X}{\frac{1}{2}}$ _____

6. $\dfrac{X}{\frac{4}{6}} = \dfrac{5}{\frac{1}{2}}$ _____

7. $\dfrac{5}{6} = \dfrac{7}{X}$ _____

8. $\dfrac{0.61}{X} = \dfrac{0.2}{0.4}$ _____

9. $\dfrac{1.5}{X} = \dfrac{15}{2.5}$ _____

10. $\dfrac{0.8}{0.9} = \dfrac{0.7}{X}$ _____

Convert to percent strength.

11. 1:500   _____

12. 5 g to 75 ml   _____

13. 1 to 10   _____

14. 15 g = 250 ml   _____

Convert to ratio strength.

15. $3\frac{1}{2}\%$ _____   16. $\frac{1}{6}\%$ _____

17. 0.02% _____   18. 8.4% _____

Solve using proportions.

19. If a 0.5% solution contains 2 grams of medication, how many milliliters of solution do you have?

20. The label on a medication reads: 15 mg per kilogram of body weight per day. How much would you give a patient weighing 35 kilograms? If the patient were given the medication three times a day, how much would you give each dose?

21. The label on a medication reads: 250 mg per tablet strength. If you are to give the patient $3\frac{1}{2}$ tablets, how many mg will the patient receive?

22. You have available a dosage strength of 8 mg in 2 ml. How many milliliters do you give a patient who needs 3 mg?

23. How many grams of medication are in 500 ml of 0.5% solution?

24. The strength available is 150 mg in 3 ml. A dosage of 250 mg has been ordered. How many milliliters do you give the patient?

25. You are to give a patient $\frac{3}{4}$ grains of medication from $1\frac{1}{2}$-grain tablets. How many tablets will you give?

Chapter 4

Apothecaries' and Household System of Measurement

This chapter explains the apothecaries' and household system of measurement. When you complete this chapter you should be able to:

a. Identify units of measure.
b. State relationships between the units of measure.
c. Accurately interpret the abbreviations and symbols that pertain to the system.
d. Chart dosages using apothecaries' measures and Roman numerals.
e. Convert units within the apothecaries' system.

4.1 Apothecaries' System

Before the Pharmaceutical Association "went metric" in 1959, apothecaries' measures were used for dispensing all medications. Today, the official system of weighing and measuring medications in the United States is the metric system. However, some institutions and physicians still use apothecaries' measures, making it necessary for a nurse to be aware of what the apothecaries' system includes. Although apothecaries' measurements continue to appear, their use should be discouraged because conversions to metric units are inaccurate.

Apothecaries' measures came into use by the apothecary, one who prepared and sold compounds for medicinal purposes. This ancient system deals only with units of weight and volume and was used exclusively to weigh and measure medications. In the old English system (see Appendix A), the smallest unit of weight is the grain (gr.). In ancient times, a millet grain or a grain of wheat was used to balance the material being weighed. The old English system of weights could be categorized according to the object to be weighed. Notice that the apothecaries' ounce is larger than the avoirdupois ounce.

English System of Weights

Troy (gold, silver, gems)	Avoirdupois (common objects)	APOTHECARIES' (medicines)
24 grain = 1 pennyweight	27.343 grains = 1 dram	**20 grains = 1 scruple**
480 grains = 1 ounce	437.5 grains = 1 ounce	**3 scruples = 1 dram**
20 pennyweights = 1 oz.	16 drams = 1 ounce	**60 grains = 1 dram**
12 ounces = 1 pound	16 ounces = 1 pound	**8 drams = 1 ounce**
		12 ounces = 1 pound

The grain is the basic unit of weight in the apothecaries' system, and the minim (M_x) is the basic unit of volume. A minim is the quantity of water (a drop) equal to the weight of a grain of wheat. Apothecaries thought it significant that the smallest unit of weight was equivalent to the smallest unit of volume, that is, a drop of water (or water-based solution) weighs one grain and has a volume of one minim. Today, this equivalence has no value because dropper sizes vary. The abbreviation for drop is **gtt.**, from the Latin word "gutta" meaning drop.

APOTHECARIES' MEASURES
60 minims = 1 dram
8 drams = 1 ounce
16 ounces = 1 pint
2 pints = 1 quart
4 quarts = 1 gallon
32 ounces = 1 quart

Because "dram" and "ounce" could mean weight or volume, we will use a different symbol to distinguish between them (see section 4.3).

4.2 *Household System*

Also part of the old English System is the "household system" of measurement. Household measures deal only with the measurement of liquid medications. They are not accurate and only approximate the amount required. Therefore, they should be avoided in the administration of medications in the hospital. Many over-the-counter (OTC) medications are dispensed this way. There is no base unit in the household system; the smallest unit is the drop.

HOUSEHOLD MEASURES
75 gtts. = 1 teaspoon
3 teaspoons = 1 tablespoon
2 tablespoons = 1 ounce
8 ounces = 1 cup
2 cups = 1 pint
2 pints = 1 quart
4 quarts = 1 gallon
32 ounces = 1 quart

Notice that a teaspoon and a dram are **not** equivalent. For practical purposes, a nurse might let 1 teaspoon = 1 dram. For example, suppose a patient is being released from the hospital with a bottle of liquid medication, and the dosage is 1 dram q.i.d. A nurse would tell this patient to take 1 teaspoon four times a day. However, when doing calculations,

avoid the conversion from dram to teaspoon whenever possible.

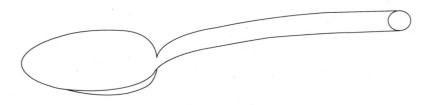

1 tsp. ≈ 1 dram

(The symbol ≈ means approximately")

4.3 Abbreviations and Symbols

Abbreviations and symbols for the apothecaries' and household system are:

Unit	Abbreviation	Symbol
gallon	gal.	C.
quart	qt.	
pint	pt.	O.
ounce	oz.	℥ or ℥
dram	dr.	ʒ or ʒ
grain	gr.	
minim	min.	♏︎ₓ
drops	gtts.	
pound	lb.	#
teaspoon	tsp.	t
tablespoon	Tbl. or Tbs. or Tbsp.	T
cup	c.	c

In all nursing situations, the symbols for ounce, dram, and minim are preferred, although you may use the abbreviation for ounce and dram for clarity. The symbols for gallon, pint, and pound are **not** used in nursing. The symbols for teaspoon and tablespoon are optional. Correct use of the English System requires periods after all abbreviations.

Note: ʒ and ʒ are handwritten; ℥ and ℥ are printed in texts.

Note: f ℥ stands for **fluid ounce**. f ʒ stands for **fluid dram**.

The profession of medicine is an ancient one, and this is reflected in its retention of some ancient language and symbolism. The use of Roman numerals **i** through **xl** are used to represent numerical amounts when medications are charted in the apothecaries' system. Both lower and upper case numerals are presented here since a nurse may occasionally see upper case, although lower case is more common.

A dot or a line is placed over the numeral for "one" to avoid confusion with the numeral L. The line may also be placed over "ii" and "ss."

Notice that $\frac{1}{2}$ has the symbol "ss." For all other fractions and mixed numbers, use Arabic numerals as they normally appear.

Roman Numerals

$\frac{1}{2}$ = ss   - - - - - - - - - - - - - -   ss is the abbreviation for "semi"; also $\overline{ss}$

1 = i or I   - - - - - - - - - - - - -   also written $\overline{\text{i}}$

2 = ii or II   - - - - - - - - - - - - -   also written $\overline{\text{ii}}$

3 = iii or III

4 = iv or IV   - - - - - - - - - - - - -   **Rule:** whenever a smaller numeral appears before a larger numeral, the smaller is subtracted. (iv means $5 - 1 = 4$)

5 = v or V

6 = vi or VI

7 = vii or VII

8 = viii or VIII

9 = ix or IX

10 = x or X

11 = xi or XI   - - - - - - - - - - - - -   **Rule:** whenever a smaller numeral appears after a larger numeral, the smaller is added. (xi means $10 + 1 = 11$)

12 = xii or XII

15 = xv or XV

20 = xx or XX

40 = xl or XL

50 = l or L

4.3 Exercises

Fill in the blanks.

	Unit of Measure	Abbreviation	Symbol
1.	gallon	_____	
2.	ounce	_____	_____
3.	dram	_____	_____
4.	minim	_____	_____
5.	tablespoon	_____	_____
6.	pound	_____	_____
7.	drops	_____	
8.	grain	_____	
9.	quart	_____	
10.	teaspoon	_____	_____
11.	pint	_____	
12.	cup	_____	

Arabic Numeral	Roman Numeral
13.	2	_____
14.	_____	v
15.	_____	viii
16.	10	_____
17.	13	_____
18.	_____	xxiv
19.	9	_____
20.	$\frac{1}{2}$	_____
21.	4	_____
22.	_____	xi
23.	6	_____
24.	15	_____
25.	_____	xix

4.4 Charted Dosages

CHARTING IN APOTHECARIES' SYSTEM
MAIN RULE: symbol or abbreviation   *then*   amount in Roman
                                                  numerals

EXCEPTIONS:

Fractions $\neq \frac{1}{2}$ symbol or abbr.   *then*   fraction in Arabic

Amount over 40   amount in Arabic   *then*   symbol or abbr.
Household   amount in Arabic   *then*   abbr.

When dosages are charted (written in prescription code) in the apothecaries' system, the amount is written in Roman numerals and appears **after** the apothecaries' unit. This rule holds true for quantities under 40 (xl). Quantities over 40 are usually expressed in Arabic numerals in front of the apothecaries' unit. For example:

Charted Dosage	Meaning
℥ ss	$\frac{1}{2}$ ounce
ℨ iii	3 drams
gr. $\frac{1}{4}$	$\frac{1}{4}$ grains
gr. $2\frac{3}{4}$	$2\frac{3}{4}$ grains
60 gr.	60 grains

Notice that Roman numerals are not used with mixed numbers (whole numbers and fractions).

The Household system uses Arabic numerals and fractions, not decimals, and the amount is written before the unit. (Note: some doctors may use Roman numerals.)

Charted Dosage	Meaning
2 tsp.	2 teaspoons
$\frac{1}{2}$ tsp.	$\frac{1}{2}$ teaspoon
ii tsp.	2 teaspoons
2 t	2 teaspoons

Small "t" is an abbreviation only for teaspoon. Abbreviate tablets as "tab."

Problems to try.

Can you read these prescriptions? Answers appear at the end of 4.4 exercises.

a.
> **℞**
> TUSSI-ORGANIDIN® ̄īī tsp.
> q. 4h. p.r.n.
>
> Dr. Well

b.
> **℞**
> AMOXIL® liquid ℥ īss
> t.i.d. for 10 days
>
> Dr. Moore

4.4   *Exercises*

State the meaning of these charted dosages.

Charted Dosage	**Meaning**
1. ℥ v t.i.d.	_____
2. ℨ iii q. 4h.	_____
3. ℳ viss b.i.d.	_____
4. gr. $\frac{3}{4}$ q.a.m.	_____
5. ℥ xx īss q. 3h.	_____
6. ̄īī tsp. q.p.m.	_____

7. $\frac{1}{2}$ pt. q.i.d. _____

8. gr. v p.r.n. _____

9. qt. $\overset{..}{\text{ii}}$ q.d. _____

10. f $\overline{\overline{3}}$ iv q.p.m. _____

11. 2 t p.c. _____

12. 1 tab b.i.d. _____

Answers to Problems to try.

a. Take 2 teaspoons every four hours when necessary   b. Take $1\frac{1}{2}$ drams three times a day for 10 days

---

Space Provided for Student Work

4.5   *Converting Units within the Apothecaries' System*

Using Factor-label Method to Convert.
Remember: Raise a fraction to higher terms by multiplying by another name for 1. The resulting fraction has the **same** value. It simply looks different. For example,

Example: $\frac{2}{3} \times \frac{4}{4} = \frac{8}{12}$ $\frac{4}{4}$ is another name for 1

You can do this with whole numbers, too.

Example: $5 \times \frac{3}{3} = \frac{5}{1} \times \frac{3}{3} = \frac{15}{3}$ 5 and $\frac{15}{3}$ are equivalent

Converting from a given unit to another unit is done in the same manner. This time the name for 1 will take the form of a conversion factor, taken from the list you are to memorize, which is summarized on the conversion card.

For example, multiplying by $\frac{12 \text{ inches}}{1 \text{ foot}}$ will not change the value of your original statement, because 12 inches = 1 foot. Therefore, we have simply multiplied by another name for 1.

Example: Express 5 feet in inches.

$$5 \text{ feet} \times \frac{12 \text{ inches}}{1 \text{ foot}} = \frac{5 \text{ feet}}{1} \times \frac{12 \text{ inches}}{1 \text{ foot}} \text{ (conversion factor)}$$

Notice that the units "feet" cancel, leaving:

$$\frac{5 \text{ feet}}{1} \times \frac{12 \text{ inches}}{1 \text{ foot}} = \frac{60 \text{ inches}}{1} = 60 \text{ inches}$$

This process of conversion is called the **factor-label method** (also called **label cancellation** or **dimensional analysis**) and is used in chemistry and science. The process gets its name because the labels "cancel" during multiplication of factors.

TO CONVERT FROM ONE UNIT TO ANOTHER:
1. write down the amount (with the units) you are converting from;
2. put an 'X' sign and draw a fraction bar;
3. put "old units" on bottom and "new units" on top;
4. find the conversion from the conversion table;
5. fill in the conversion numbers with their respective units;
6. solve.

$$\text{amount} \times \frac{\text{new units}}{\text{old units}} = \text{new units}$$

Example: 5 Tbsp. = _____ drams.

Convert tablespoons to drams. The conversion card states that 1 Tbsp. = 4 drams. Tablespoons are the "old units" and drams are the "new units." Following the steps gives:

$$5 \text{ Tbsp.} \times \frac{4 \text{ drams}}{1 \text{ Tbsp.}} = 20 \text{ drams (the conversion was 4 dr.} = 1 \text{ T)}$$

Remember: make sure the units will "cancel" correctly. It they do not, then you know you have set up the problem incorrectly.

Example: 12 t = _____ T

We know that 1 T = 3 t. The set up looks like this:

$$12 \text{ t} \times \frac{1 \text{ T}}{3 \text{ t}} = \frac{12 \text{ T}}{3} = 4 \text{ T}$$

Example: 2 dr. = _____ ♏x

$$2 \text{ drams} \times \frac{60 \text{ ♏x}}{1 \text{ dram}} = \frac{120 \text{ ♏x}}{1} = 120 \text{ ♏x}$$

Example: $1\frac{1}{2}$ gal. = _____ oz.

We know that 32 oz. = 1 qt. and that 4 qt. = 1 gal. We have no direct conversion from gallons to ounces and will have to use two conversion factors. First set up the problem using only the units, then fill in the numbers.

$$\text{gal.} \times \frac{\text{qt.}}{\text{gal.}} \times \frac{\text{oz.}}{\text{qt.}} = \text{oz.}$$

$$1.5 \, \cancel{\text{gal.}} \times \frac{4 \, \cancel{\text{qt.}}}{1 \, \cancel{\text{gal.}}} \times \frac{32 \, \text{oz.}}{1 \, \cancel{\text{qt.}}} = 192 \, \text{oz.}$$

The first conversion canceled out the old units and the second conversion yielded the new units.

Example: $1\frac{1}{2}$ oz. = _____ dr.

Fractions can be dealt with in several ways:

$$1\frac{1}{2} \, \text{oz.} \times \frac{8 \, \text{drams}}{1 \, \text{ounce}} =$$

$$1.5 \, \cancel{\text{oz.}} \times \frac{8 \, \text{drams}}{1 \, \cancel{\text{ounce}}} = \frac{12}{1} = 12 \, \text{drams}$$

or

$$\frac{3}{2} \, \cancel{\text{oz.}} \times \frac{8 \, \text{drams}}{1 \, \cancel{\text{ounce}}} = \frac{24}{2} = 12 \, \text{drams}$$

It is important to stay within the apothecaries' system, as is evident in the following problem. The second calculation is correct, and the first is inaccurate.

Example: 4 oz. = _____ pt.

Wrong way: $4 \, \text{oz.} \times \frac{30 \, \text{ml}}{1 \, \text{oz.}} \times \frac{1 \, \text{pt.}}{500 \, \text{ml}} = \frac{120}{500} \, \text{pt.} = 0.24 \, \text{pt.}$

Right way: $4 \, \text{oz.} \times \frac{1 \, \text{pt.}}{16 \, \text{oz.}} = \frac{4}{16} \, \text{pt.} = \frac{1}{4} \, \text{pt.} = 0.25 \, \text{pt.}$

If there is a direct conversion on the conversion table, use it. Do not go from one system to another then back to the original system. Stay in the same system whenever possible.

Problems to try. Answers to these problems appear at the end of 4.5 exercises.

a. $\frac{1}{2}$ oz. = _____ $\mathfrak{m}_x$ b. 120 grains = _____ oz.

Using Proportions to Convert

Recall that a proportion is a statement that two fractions are equal. To solve a proportion for a missing number, set the "cross products" equal. The simplest way to set up a proportion is to use the conversion unit as one side of the proportion, and the ordered amount on the other side.

Example: 2 oz. = _____ Tbsp.

The conversion (1 oz. = 2 Tbsp.) is on one side of the proportion.

$$\frac{2 \text{ oz.}}{X \text{ Tbsp.}} = \frac{1 \text{ oz.}}{2 \text{ Tbsp.}}$$ set up the proportion

$$X = 2(2) = 4 \text{ Tbsp.}$$ cross multiply

Example: $\frac{1}{2}$ dr. = _____ $\mathfrak{m}_x$

$$\frac{\frac{1}{2} \text{ dr.}}{X \, \mathfrak{m}_x} = \frac{1 \text{ dr.}}{60 \, \mathfrak{m}_x}$$ set up the proportion

$$X = \frac{1}{2}(60) = 30 \, \mathfrak{m}_x$$ cross multiply

Problems to try. Answers to these problems appear at the end of 4.5 exercises.

c. $\frac{1}{2}$ oz. = _____ dr.

d. 180 $\mathfrak{m}_x$ = _____ dr.

e. 24 dr. = _____ oz.

If (on the job) you have worked a conversion and the answer consistently seems unlikely, follow these steps for remediation:

    a. Rework the problem, rechecking the conversion units.
    b. Ask a peer to work the problem.
    c. Check with a pharmacist.

4.5   Exercises

Convert each unit as indicated. Show your work. Chart the answers to the first 10 problems. Do **not** chart answers to 11–20.

1. gr. xxx = ℥ _____

2. gr. 100 = ℥ _____

3. ℥ xxiv = ℥ _____

4. ℥ ss = ℥ _____

5. dr. īss = ♏︎ₓ _____

6. ℥ T = gr. _____

7. ℥ ivss = _____ Tbsp.

8. ℥ īī = _____ Tbsp.

9. f ℥ $\frac{1}{6}$ = _____ ♏︎ₓ

10. ℥ $\frac{1}{8}$ = gr. _____

11. 3 pt. = _____ qt.

12. 4 T = _____ t

13. 5 gal. = _____ pt.

14. $\frac{1}{2}$ gal. = _____ oz.

15. 3 pt. = _____ oz.

16. 6 pt. = _____ gal.

17. 10 qt. = _____ gal.

18. $\frac{1}{2}$ qt. = _____ oz.

19. 24 dr. = _____ oz.

20. 2 dr. = _____ minims

Answers to Problems to try.

a. 240 minims   b. $\frac{1}{4}$ ounce   c. 4 drams   d. 3 drams   e. 3 ounces

4.6   Word Problems

Remember: Total medication = Amount per tablet × Number of tablets

Number of tablets = Total medication ÷ Amount per tablet

Read the problem until you understand what is given and what must be found. When you get the answer, go back, and read the problem to see if your answer makes sense.

Example: Ordered: gr. x

Available: $2\frac{1}{2}$ grain tablets

Give _____ tablets

10 grains ÷ $2\frac{1}{2}$ grain = 4 tablets

Example: The doctor orders Elixir ℥ iv q.i.d. How many ounces is the patient getting daily?   _____

4 drams 4 times per day = 4 × 4 = 16 drams per day

16 drams × $\frac{1 \text{ ounce}}{8 \text{ drams}}$ = 2 ounces per day

4.6   Exercises

1.   Ordered: gr. v
     Medication on hand: $2\frac{1}{2}$ grain tablets
     Give _____ tablets.

2.   Ordered: gr. ss
     Medication on hand: $\frac{1}{6}$ grain tablets
     Give _____ tablets.

3. Ordered: gr. vi
   Medication on hand: 12 grain tablets
   Give _____ tablets.

4. You need solution for 10 irrigations during the day. If you need 1 pint for each irrigation, how many quarts should you prepare?

5. An infant receives 2 oz. of formula q.3h. How many quarts of formula has he taken in a three-day period?

6. An infant receives 4 oz. of formula q.4h. How many quarts of formula has he taken in a four-day period?

7. A patient receives 1 tsp. MAALOX® q.i.d. If MAALOX® comes in 6 oz. bottles, how many bottles are needed for a two-week supply?

8. The doctor orders MAALOX® ℥ss q.6h. If MAALOX® comes in 6 oz. bottles, how many bottles are needed for a ten-day supply?

9. The doctor orders elixir ℥ ii t.i.d. How many ounces is the patient getting daily?

10. A patient is given 2 ounces of medication q.6h. for 3 days. How many total drams is this?

11. The doctor orders QUELIDRINE® syrup T̄ tsp. q.i.d. How long will a four-ounce bottle last?

12. If a patient is given 1 tsp. of TUSSAR® SF syrup q.4h. for 12 days, how many ounces have been given?

13.   If you give a patient 3 tablets of strength 5 gr. per tab., how many total grains of medication did he receive?

14.   If you give a patient $\frac{1}{2}$ ounce of solution of strength 30 gr. per oz., how many total grains of medication did he receive?

15.   If you give a patient $1\frac{1}{2}$ ounces of solution of strength 40 gr. per oz., how many total grains of medication did he receive?

_____

Space Provided for Student Work

_____

Chapter 4 Test

Write in the symbols as they would be charted.

1. eight minims   _____

2. five drams   _____

3. three and one-half ounces   _____

4. one and one-half fluid drams   _____

5. ten grains   _____

6. two tablets   _____

7. two teaspoons   _____

Translate into words.

8. ℥ īss q.i.d.   _____

9. ℥ iii q.a.m.   _____

10. ʒ iv b.i.d.   _____

11. qt. Ī q.d.   _____

12. f ʒ   p.r.n.   _____

13. gr. $\frac{1}{10}$ q.d.   _____

Convert to the indicated unit.

14.   12 drams = _____ ounces

15.   6 quarts = _____ gallons

16.   120 minims = _____ drams

17.   1 cup = _____ tablespoons

18.   3 pints = _____ ounces

19.   2 liquid ounces = _____ liquid drams

20.   90 grains = _____ drams

21. $1\frac{1}{2}$ qts. = _____ ounces

Solve.

22.   If a child drinks three 8-oz glasses of milk each day, how many quarts should be available for a three-day supply?

23.   A patient takes 1 tsp. of TUSSI-ORGANIDIN® q.4h. for two days. How many ounces has he taken?

24. A nurse is preparing saline solution for six irrigations during the day. If each irrigation requires 16 ounces, how many 1-gallon containers are needed to contain the solution?

25. An infant is given 8 ounces of formula every 4 hours. If the formula is available in quart cans, what is the least number of cans needed for a five-day supply?

26. EES® comes in one pint bottles. How many $\frac{1}{4}$-ounce doses can you get out of a bottle?

27. A nurse gives one ounce of Milk of Magnesia q.d. for two weeks. How many ounces are left in a 1-pint bottle?

28. The doctor orders KAON® Elixir $\overline{\dot{\text{I}}}$ Tbsp. b.i.d. after morning and evening meals. How many days will 1 pint of medication last?

29. An infant is given 6 ounces of formula every 4 hours. If the formula is available in quart cans, what is the least number of cans needed for a four-day supply?

30. Read Appendix A.

Chapter 5

Metric System of Measurement

This chapter explains the metric system of measurement. When you complete this chapter you should be able to:

a. Identify and/or list metric units of length, volume, weight and temperature.
b. State relationships between the units of measure.
c. Interpret abbreviations used in the metric system.
d. Convert from one metric measure to another.

5.1 Introduction, Base Units, and Prefixes

As health care professionals, you need to be at ease with the metric system, because most medications are dispensed metrically and many hospitals are beginning to use metric weights, temperature, and digital time. The metric system began in France in 1790 (see Appendix A for more history), and is the most widely used system of measurement in the world. The United States is virtually the only country that does not use the metric system as its primary system of measurement. The value of the metric system lies in its simplicity, accuracy, and flexibility. The correct name for the metric system is "**SI**," which stands for "**International System of Units**." There are only seven base units in SI (compared to 85 in the English system). They are:

> length = meter (m)
> mass (weight) = kilogram (kg)
> time = second (s)
> temperature = degrees Celsius (°C)

> amount of substance = mole (mol)
> electrical current = ampere (A)
> luminous intensity = candela (cd)

> volume (a related unit) = liter (ℓ or L)

The metric system is a decimal system of measurement, while the apothecaries' and household systems are fractional systems. Decimals are easier and faster to use than fractions. To convince yourself of this, *try timing yourself as you mark the ruler measures that follow on pages* 121 *and* 122 Most people require twice as long to mark the English ruler than the metric ruler, even if they have never seen a metric ruler.

BASIC RULES OF THE METRIC SYSTEM:
1. **when in doubt over pronunciation, accent the first syllable;**
2. **there are no periods after metric abbreviations;**
3. **metric units are not capitalized except for Celsius;**
4. **unit symbols are never made plural; 5 mm not 5 mms;**
5. **leave a space between number and symbol: 10 cm not 10cm (Exception: when charting dosages, the space is purposely omitted to avoid tampering with dosage amounts on prescriptions.)**

The English system, has a different name for larger or smaller measures, such as inch, foot, yard, mile. The metric system, uses only one base unit, such as meter, with prefixes to make larger or smaller measures: i.e., **milli**meter, **centi**meter, **kilo**meter. The metric system is a system of prefixes. A complete list of prefixes can be found in Appendix A.

Metric Prefixes

Multiple in decimal form	Power of 10	Prefix	Symbol	Pronunciation	Meaning
1000	10^3	kilo	k	kĭl′ ō	one thousand times base
100	10^2	hecto	h	hĕk′ tō	one hundred times base
10	10^1	deka	da	dĕk′ ă	ten times base
1	10^0	**base unit**			
0.1	10^{-1}	deci	d	dĕs′ ĭ	one tenth times base
0.01	10^{-2}	centi	c	sĕnt′ ĭ	one hundred times base
0.001	10^{-3}	milli	m	mĭl′ ĭ	one thousandth times base
0.000001	10^{-6}	micro	μ	mĭ′ krō	one millionth times base

Charted Dosages

CHARTING IN THE METRIC SYSTEM

MAIN RULE: Amount as a decimal *then* **metric abbreviation**

DO NOT leave a space between the number and the abbreviation.

Examples: three-fourths gram   0.75g
               five and a half centimeters 5.5cm
               twenty milligrams   20mg
               one-half milliliter   0.5ml

In charting dosages, it is advisable to omit the space to avoid possible tampering with medication dosages. When doing calculations in the metric system, leave the space for clarity in your computations.

5.1   Exercises

Name the basic units in the metric system.

1. basic unit of length: _____

2. basic unit of time: _____

3. basic unit of weight (mass): _____

4. basic unit of temperature: _____

5. related unit of volume: _____

Name the prefix by name and by symbol.

6. one-thousandth of base unit: _____   symbol: _____

7. one-hundredth of base unit: _____   symbol: _____

8. one-thousand times base unit: _____   symbol: _____

9. one-millionth of base unit: _____   symbol: _____

10. one-tenth of base unit: _____   symbol: _____

Write the correct abbreviation.

11. 2.5 milliliters _____

12. 5.0 centimeters _____

13. 50 milligrams _____

14. 200 micrograms _____

15. 1.5 kilometers _____

16. 300 millimeters _____

How would the following be charted:

17. two and one-half milliliters three times a day   _____

18. 50 milligrams at bedtime   _____

19. $\frac{1}{4}$ of a gram in the morning   _____

20. two liters per day   _____

21. 600 micrograms twice a day   _____

22. infant length: fifty-two and one-half centimeters   _____

23. patient weight: sixty-two kilograms   _____

24. 150 milliliters every six hours   _____

25. $\frac{1}{2}$ of a gram every four hours   _____

State the meaning of these charted dosages.

26. 2.5cc IM   t.i.d.   _____

27. 30ml   q.a.m.   _____

28. 250μg/ml   q.p.m.   _____

29. 5ml   q.3h.   _____

30. 0.375g   p.r.n.   _____

31. 500μg/ml   q.h.   _____

Space Provided for Student Work

Ruler Reading Test

$\dfrac{7}{8}$"

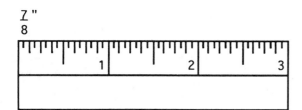

$4\dfrac{3}{4}$"

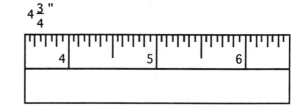

$8\dfrac{3}{8}$"

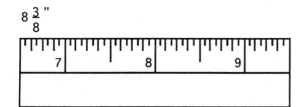

$11\dfrac{1}{16}$"

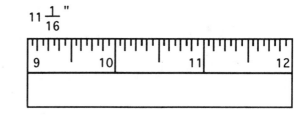

$4\dfrac{1}{4}$"

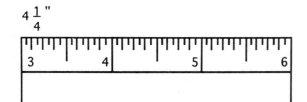

$1\dfrac{3}{4}$"

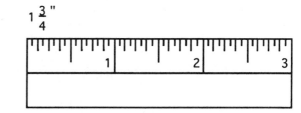

$6\dfrac{5}{16}$"

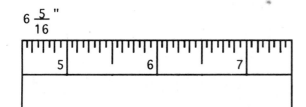

$10\dfrac{5}{8}$"

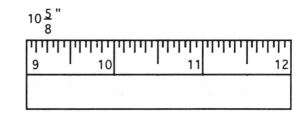

$2\dfrac{9}{16}$"

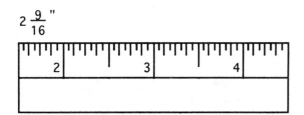

$9\dfrac{13}{16}$"

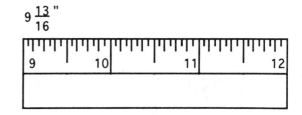

Ruler Reading Test

0.3
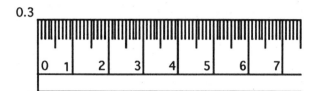

5.1
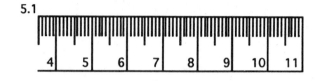

6.2
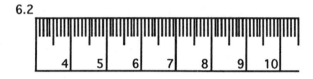

8.8
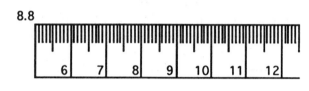

23.9

2.7
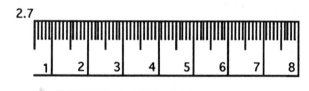

17.0

12.4

28.5
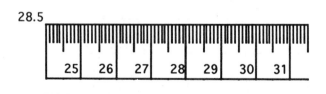

42.6
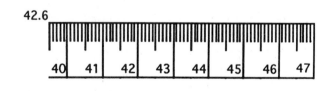

5.2 Metric Length

The **basic unit of length** in the metric system is the **meter**. The word "meter" comes from the Greek word "metron" meaning "to measure." The meter was originally defined as a portion of the earth's circumference, but now it is defined as a certain number of wavelengths of light (see Appendix A for a more precise definition).

A meter is a yard plus a little extra.

if this were a yard

this would be a meter

millimeter -

if this were a mile

centimeter ——

if this would be a kilometer

inch ————

Instead of using miles, use kilometers; instead of yards, use meters; instead of inches, use centimeters. For very small measurements, use millimeters. You may find it helpful to learn small metric units of length by comparison to familiar objects. A millimeter is about the width of the wire on a paper clip. A centimeter is the width of a paper clip, and a decimeter is about the length of three paper clips lined up end-to-end. The ruler test on the previous page corresponds to centimeters.

1 decimeter = 10 centimeters

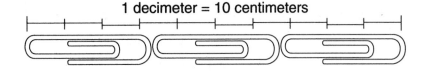

A nurse will use metric length in the following situations:

Unit	Symbol	Use
centimeter	cm	tracheotomy tube orthopedic apparatus anatomical part measurement height of patient dilatation of cervix during labor
millimeter	mm	anatomical measurement dressings ostomy measurement tubing needle size iodoform packing
square centimeter	cm^2	surgical preparation (area size) pharmaceutical ointment decubitus protective device

Needle size is based on the standard wire gauge number of the diameter of the shaft, suffixed by the letter G, and followed by the multiplication sign and the length, in inches, of the shaft. Metric equivalents are also used.

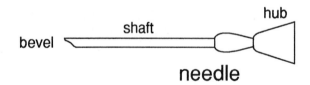

needle

Designated Size

Non-metric (in.)	Metric (mm)
26 G × 5/8	0.45 × 16
25 G × 3/4	0.50 × 20
24 G × 3/4	0.55 × 20
23 G × 1	0.60 × 25
22 G × 1 1/4	0.70 × 32
21 G × 1 1/2	0.80 × 38
20 G × 1 1/2	0.90 × 38
19 G × 1 5/8	1.00 × 41
18 G × 1 1/2	1.20 × 38
15 G × 1 1/2	1.80 × 38

5.2   Exercises

Use the metric ruler to measure the following lines.

1.   _____

2.   _____

3.   _____

4.   _____

5.   _____

6.   In orthopedics, a patient is checked for scoliosis by carefully measuring his height when sitting and subtracting the height of the chair. If a patient measures 130 cm sitting, and the chair seat is 42 cm high, what measurement is recorded as the length of the patient's spine (plus head)?

7.   How long is the patient's spine (plus head) if sitting height is 142 cm and the height of the chair is 28.5 cm?

Chart the following using the metric system.

8.   one-half of a centimeter   _____

9.   an infant measures forty-four and a half centimeters   _____

10.   length of Foley catheter is nineteen and a half centimeters   _____

11.   tubing is four and a half millimeters   _____

12.   six and three-tenths centimeters   _____

In what metric unit are the following measured?

13.   needle size   _____

14.   length of crutches   _____

15. width of Foley catheter   _____

16. distance to place heat lamp from patient   _____

17. newborn infant's height   _____

18. surgical preparation (area size)   _____

19. tracheotomy tube   _____

Without using a ruler (do **not** use one) try to draw a line that is:

20.   1 cm long

21.   5 cm long

22.   10 cm long

23.   1 mm long

24.   85 mm long

25.   20 mm long

5.3   *Metric Volume*

The liter is **not** a base unit in the metric system. Because volume is related to length, **the liter is called a related unit**. If you had a cube that measured 10 cm × 10 cm × 10 cm, the volume would be 1000 cubic centimeters, or a liter.

$$1 \text{ liter} = 1000 \text{ cm}^3 = 1000 \text{ cc}$$

In medicine, cubic centimeter is abbreviated cc instead of cm³. The following picture is the actual size of a liter. Although you cannot tell by looking at the picture, the *liter is only slightly larger than a quart.*

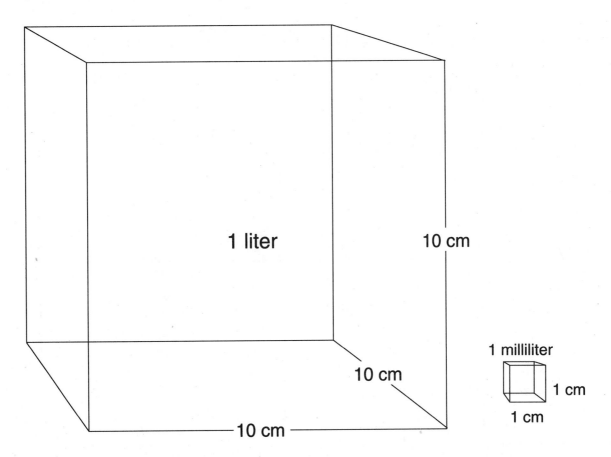

A cube that measures 1 cm × 1 cm × 1 cm is a cubic centimeter. Since there are 1000 cm³ (or 1000 cc) in one liter, and since one-thousandth of a liter is called a milliliter, **1 cc = 1 ml**. The *milliliter is much smaller than a teaspoon.* In fact, it takes 5 ml to make one teaspoon.

Use liters instead of quarts, and use milliliters instead of cups, ounces, and teaspoons.

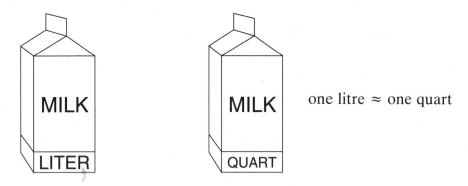

one litre ≈ one quart

To convert from milliliters to liters, determine what part of a liter is given.

Example: 200 ml = _____ ℓ

200 ml out of 1000 ml   is $\frac{200}{1000}$ ℓ   or   0.200 ℓ

A nurse will use metric volume in the following situations:

Unit	Symbol	Use
cubic centimeter or milliliter (used interchangeably)	cc (or cm³) ml	I & O measurement IV fluid catheter—irrigation amount catheter—balloon size oxygen administration IM injection (fluid in syringe) pharmaceutical measurement stock solution hypothermia blanket fluid
liter	ℓ	I & O measurement oxygen administration IV fluid pharmaceutical measurement
milliliter per minute	ml/min.	fluid consumption ratio—IV irrigation gavages

Remember:

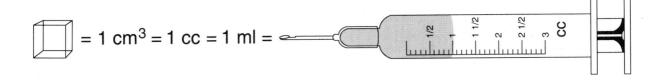

Notice that each mark on this syringe represents 0.1 cc.

5.3   *Exercises*

---

1. A liter is about the same volume as a _____

2. A cubic centimeter is one-fifth the size of a _____

Remembering that 1000 cc = 1000 ml = 1 liter, change each of the following to the indicated measure.

3. 2 liters = _____ ml

4. 30 cc =   _____ ml

5. 500 cc = _____ liter

6. 250 ml = _____ liter

7. 100 cc = _____ liter

8. $\frac{1}{4}$ liter = _____ cc
    How should $\frac{1}{4}$ liter be correctly written? _____

9. 0.5 liter = _____ ml

10. 0.25 liter = _____ cm^3

11. 250 cm^3 = _____ ml

12. 2500 cm^3 = _____ ℓ

13. 600 cm^3 = _____ cc

14. 3000 ml = _____ ℓ

15. 25 cc = _____ cm^3 = _____ ml

16. 0.25 liter = _____ cc

17. 2 liters = _____ cm^3

Matching:

_____ 18. volume of a teaspoon   A. 1 ml

_____ 19. volume of a glass of milk   B. 5 ml

_____ 20. volume of a gallon of milk   C. 250 ml

_____ 21. volume of a sugar cube   D. 4 liters

_____ 22. volume of a large auto gas tank   E. 80 liters

Choose milliliter (ml) or liter (ℓ) to answer each of the following.

23. I have 250 _____ of coffee in my cup.

24. My medicine bottle holds 75 _____ of medicine.

25. You should drink 2 _____ of water daily.

26. The bathtub holds 80 _____ of water.

27. Please add 2 _____ of medicine to the IV fluids.

28. The flower vase holds 300 _____ of water.

29. The syringe holds 5 _____ of medicine.

How would the following be charted?

30. one-half of a cubic centimeter _____

31. two and one-half cubic centimeters _____

32. three-fourths of a milliliter _____

33. 1000 milliliters _____

34. 1 liter _____

In what metric unit(s) is each of the following measured?

35. IM injections _____

36. stock solutions _____

37. output measurements _____

38. P.O. fluid intake _____

39. irrigation amount for catheter _____

40. oral medication _____

41. oxygen administration _____

42. capacity of flask of 5% dextrose/water for IV _____

43. IV solution _____

5.4   *Metric Mass*

The **basic unit of weight, or mass**, in the metric system is the **kilogram**. (Until 1960, the gram was the basic unit.) The kilogram is the only base unit that contains a prefix. (see History of Metric System in Appendix A.) However, **gram is the unit to which prefixes are added**.

$$\boxed{\textbf{1 kilogram = 1000 grams}}$$

In the metric system, volume and mass have a special relationship. At sea level, at 4° Celsius, **1 milliliter of water weighs 1 gram, and 1 liter of water weighs 1 kilogram**. *This is the definition of the kilogram and the gram.*

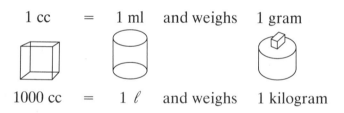

The most commonly used units of mass are gram and kilogram. When speaking of large quantities, such as a large truck, the unit of metric ton (1000 kg) is used; and when speaking of very small quantities, such as the various ingredients of a pill, the units of milligram and possibly microgram are used.

Examples of metric weight:
    a dry teabag has a mass of 2 grams;
    a medium egg has a mass of 50 grams;
    most IV's weigh 1 kilogram (1 liter solution bags);
    a newborn baby weighs between 2.5–4 kilograms;
    average adult weight is considered to be 70 kilograms.

In medicine, microgram is often abbreviated mcg instead of μg. Some nurses abbreviate gram as Gm (or gm) to avoid confusion with grain (gr.). Mathematicians discourage this practice since it does not follow the recommendations of the National Bureau of Weights and Measures.

A nurse will use metric mass in the following situations:

Unit	Symbol	Use
micrograms	μg	pharmaceutical measurement
milligrams	mg	pharmaceutical measurement
gram	g	dietary instruction body mass of infant pharmaceutical measurement
kilogram	kg	body mass (children & adults) orthopedic traction weight

5.4   Exercises

Complete each statement below with the appropriate unit selected from among kilogram (kg), gram (g), and milligram (mg).

1. An aspirin tablet has a mass of 324 _____.

2. A new tube of chapstick has a mass of 5 _____.

3. A big newborn baby might have a mass of 5.3 _____.

4. Average adult weight is considered to be a mass of 70 _____.

5. A Bic pen has a mass of 7 _____.

6. A raisin has a mass of 330 _____.

7. Two pain pills might have a mass of 600 _____.

8. A pair of eyeglasses has a mass of 40 _____.

9. A bucket of water has a mass of 12 _____.

10. A sheet of paper has a mass of 3 _____.

For each of the following, assume volume and weight refer to water at 4°C.

11.   15 cc weigh _____ grams

12.   250 ml weigh _____ grams

13.   4 liters weigh _____ kilograms

14.   2 liters weigh _____ grams

15.   3000 ml weigh _____ kilograms

16.   1.5 liter = _____ ml and weighs _____ grams

17.   2500 ml weigh _____ kilograms

18.   72 grams is the weight of _____ cc

19.   0.5 grams is the weight of _____ cc

20.   500 grams is the weight of _____ cc

21.   500 grams is the weight of _____ liter

22.   1500 grams is the weight of _____ liters

How would the following be charted?

23.   five and two-tenths kilograms _____

24.   seven and one-half gram _____

25.   three-fourths kilogram _____

26.   twenty-five milligrams _____

In what unit would each of the following be measured?

27.   body mass of a child _____

28.   pharmaceutical measurements _____

5.5 Metric Time

The **basic unit of time** in the metric system is the **second**. Many hospitals use the 24-hour clock. Also, as a result of the metric influence, elementary school teachers are teaching "digital clock" reading (hour followed by minutes).

In health care, time is always given as hour followed by minutes.

wrong: a quarter of 2
correct: 1:45 A.M.

wrong: half past 3
correct: 3:30 P.M.

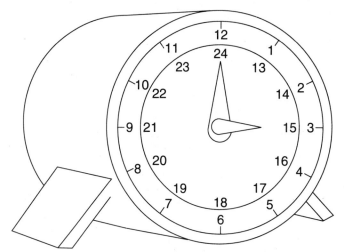

Seconds are usually divided into 10th's (as on a stop watch).

Example: 20.4 seconds

Time is written this way using a 24-hour clock:

0000	meaning	12:00 Midnight
0001		12:01 A.M.
0100		1:00 A.M.
0600		6:00 A.M.
1200		12:00 Noon
1201		12:01 P.M.
1500		3:00 P.M.
1830		6:30 P.M.
2112		9:12 P.M.
2359		11:59 P.M. Notice:
2400		12:00 Midnight 0000 = 2400

To convert to the 24-hour clock, add 1200 to a P.M. time.

Example: 5:00 P.M. is written 500 + 1200 = 1700

Dates

You are encouraged to write dates in chronological order (day, month, year; or year, month, day).

wrong:	March 13, 1984	wrong:	7/21/90
correct:	13 March 1984	correct:	90 · 7 · 21

5.5   *Exercises*

State the time of day in customary terms:

Example: 1315 = 1:15 P.M.

1.   1430 = _____

2.   0600 = _____

3.   1300 = _____

4.   1815 = _____

5.   2130 = _____

6.   1545 = _____

7.   0715 = _____

8.   0245 = _____

9.   2359 = _____

10.   2230 = _____

Write these dates correctly (in chronological order).

11.   March 15, 1992   _____

12.   January 12, 1989   _____

13.   October 3, 1990   _____

14.   May 28, 1991   _____

15.   September 9, 1988   _____

5.6 Metric Temperature

The Kelvin, symbol K, is really the basic unit of temperature in the metric system. However, **Celsius temperature**, symbol **C**, is more commonly used as a **base unit** and for ordinary use, such as for daily weather reporting, and room, bath, and body temperatures. Kelvin temperatures are used in scientific work. The lowest point on the Kelvin scale is called absolute zero—there are no negative readings. Water freezes at 273°K. A 1-degree change in Kelvin equals 1 degree of change Celsius.

$$°K = °C + 273°$$

On the Celsius scale (named for Anders Celsius, the Swedish astronomer who first devised it in 1742), water freezes at 0°C and boils at 100°C. You can compare temperatures measured on a Celsius thermometer with the Fahrenheit thermometer below. Here is a rule of thumb for quickly comparing air temperatures measured in Celsius:

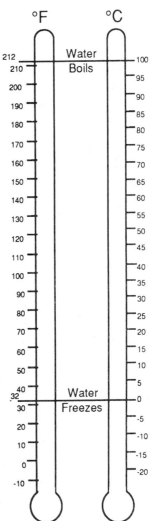

Temperatures beginning with a 3 = extremely hot
Temperatures beginning with a 2 = pleasantly warm
Temperatures beginning with a 1 = pleasantly cool
Temperatures between 0 and 10 = cold
Temperatures below 0 = below freezing
Temperatures below −20 = extremely cold

Four reference temperatures to remember are:

> 0°C = water freezes
> 20°–22°C = room temperature
> 37°C = normal body temperature
> 100°C = water boils

Metric temperature is sometimes referred to in degrees "centigrade." The word "centigrade" historically refers to angle degrees, not temperature degrees. This text recommends using **Celsius** for metric temperature.

A nurse will use metric temperature in the following situations:

Clinical thermometer in degrees Celsius

Dangerous fever	41°C
High Fever	39°C
Low grade fever	38°C
Normal temp	37°C
Subnormal temp	36°C
Abnormal temp	35°C

Bath thermometer in degrees Celsius

Hot water bottle temp	44°C
Sitz bath temp	43°C
Bed bath temp	41°C
Tub bath temp	41°C

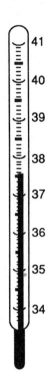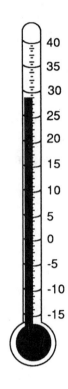

Weather thermometer in degrees Celsius

Freezing point	0°C
Room Temperature	20°–22°C

5.6   Exercises

Match the best answers together.

_____	1. Oven temp to bake a cake	A.	−273°C
_____	2. A hot day in July in Illinois	B.	−25°C
_____	3. Sweater weather	C.	−5°C
_____	4. Temperature to go ice skating	D.	15°C
_____	5. Absolute zero	E.	30°C
_____	6. High fever	F.	40°C
_____	7. Coldest day in winter in Illinois	G.	200°C

State the four reference temperatures in Celsius.

8.   Water freezes at   _____°C

9.   Room temp is   _____°C

10. Normal body temp is   _____°C

11. Water boils at   _____°C

Complete the following:

12. Dangerous fever is   _____°C

13. High fever is   _____°C

14. Low grade fever is   _____°C

15. Subnormal temp is   _____°C

16. Abnormal temp is   _____°C

Read each of the thermometers in Celsius.

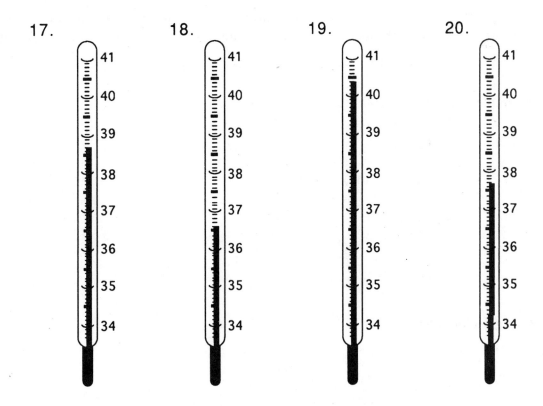

17.   18.   19.   20.

5.7   Internal Metric Conversions

Converting within the metric system can be done using the same procedures as converting within the apothecaries system. Those procedures are the **proportion method** and the **factor-label method** (see section 4.5). In addition, converting within the metric system can quickly be done using the Metric Conversion Chart.

Metric Conversion Chart
kilo-, hecto-, deka-   meter liter   deci-, centi-, milli- gram
Move the decimal point the same number of places and in the same direction the unit moves on the chart.

To use the Metric Conversion Chart, move the decimal point the same number of places and in the same direction the unit moves on the chart.

In general, to change from smaller to larger units, move the decimal point to the left; to change from larger to smaller units, move the decimal point to the right.

Note: There are two unnamed prefix units of 10 between milli and micro. When converting between these two prefixes, remember to add two additional decimal places.

Example: Change 300 g to kg.

Using a proportion

$$\frac{300 \text{ g}}{X \text{ kg}} = \frac{1000 \text{ g}}{1 \text{ kg}}$$

$$1000 \text{ X} = 300$$

$$X = \frac{300}{1000} = 0.3 \text{ kg}$$

Using factor-label method

$$300 \text{ g} \times \frac{1 \text{ kg}}{1000 \text{ g}} = \frac{300}{1000} \text{ kg} = 0.3 \text{ kg}$$

Using the Metric Conversion Chart

To go from grams to kilograms on the chart, move left three places.

300 g = 0.300 kg

Problems to try. Answers to these problems appear at the end of 5.7 exercises.

a. 480 ml = _____ ℓ

b. 0.5 kg = _____ g

c. 3 m = _____ cm

d. 2 mg = _____ μg

5.7   *Exercises*

Convert each of the following to the indicated measure.

1. 83 g = _____ mg

2. 3000 g = _____ kg

3. 5.6 kg = _____ g

4. 250 ml = _____ ℓ

5. 2 ℓ = _____ ml

6. 150 mg = _____ g

7. 5000 mg = _____ kg

8. 20 mg = _____ μg

9. 165 cm = _____ m

10. 35 mm = _____ cm

11. 1.80 m = _____ cm

12. 3600 m = _____ km

13. 150 μg = _____ mg

14. 0.375 g = _____ mg

15. 225 mg = _____ g

16. 50 mg = _____ g

17. 0.2 g = _____ mg

18. 375 ml = _____ ℓ

19. 0.75 ℓ = _____ ml

20. 1500 ml = _____ ℓ

21. 1.2 ℓ = _____ ml

22. 0.675 kg = _____ g

23. 3500 μg = _____ g

24. 0.02 km = _____ cm

25. 0.08 kg = _____ g

26. 4500 ml = _____ ℓ

27. 0.08 g = _____ μg

28. 31 cm^3 = _____ ml

29. 1200 cc = _____ ℓ

30. 0.5 ℓ = _____ cm^3

Answers to Problems to try.

a. 0.480 ℓ b. 500 g   c. 300 cm   d. 2000 μg

5.8 Word Problems

Remember: Total medication = Amount per tablet × Number of tablets

Number of tablets = Total medication ÷ Amount per tablet

Read the problem until you understand what is given and what must be found. When you get the answer, go back, and read the problem to see if your answer makes sense.

Example: Ordered: 0.5 g of a medication
Available: tablets containing 0.25 g each
Give _____ tablets

0.5 g ÷ 0.25 g = 2 tablets

Example: If a patient is to receive 1200 mg of medication per day to be given in divided doses t.i.d. How much is given for each dose?

1200 mg ÷ 3 doses = 400 mg per dose

Example: Ordered: 1 g of a medication
Available: tablets labeled 250 mg each
Give _____ tablets.

1 g ÷ 250 mg = 1000 mg ÷ 250 mg = 4 tablets

5.8 Exercises

1. Ordered: 0.75 g of a medication
   Available: tablets containing 0.25 g each
   Give _____ tablets.

2. Ordered: 1 g KEFLEX® (cephalexin)
   Available: capsules labeled 500 mg

   Give _____ capsules

3.   Ordered: 0.25 g of a medication
     Available: tablets labeled 0.5 g
     Give _____ tablets.

4.   Ordered: 0.6 mg digitalis
     Available: 0.24 mg tabs
     Give _____ tablets.

5.   Ordered: 150 mg of a medication
     Available: 100 mg tablets
     Give _____ tablets.

6.   If a patient is given 5.0 ml four times a day, she is receiving _____ cc of medication daily.

7.   A patient receives a total of 1500 mg of medication daily. How much is given for each dose if given q.i.d.?

8.   You are applying NITRO-BID® ointment, and 1 inch = 15 mg of nitroglycerin. If you apply $2\frac{1}{2}$ inches, how many milligrams did you apply?

9.   The M.D. orders EES®, 400 mg per day b.i.d. For a b.i.d. dosage, give half the daily dose q.12h. How much would you give for each dose?

10. A patient is to receive 0.5 g of a medication. The tablets are available in 5, 50, 500, or 5000 mg strengths. Which tablet do you use?

11. The medication ordered comes in 50 mg tablets (unscored). If 175 mg q.d. are ordered, how many would you give? (Note: in a situation such as this, you should check with the doctor or pharmacist before administering any amount)

12.   A patient receives DILANTIN® in 50 mg tablets. The order reads 2 tab b.i.d. How many would be needed for a week's supply?

13.   If 2 ml of blood contains 2.3 grams hemoglobin, how much hemoglobin would you expect to find in 5 ml of blood?

14.   You are to give a patient one-half of a vial. If the vial contains 2.5 ml, how many milliliters will you give to the patient?

15.   If you give 3 tablets of glycerol trinitrate, each containing 0.15 mg, how many milligrams have you given? How many micrograms is this?

Space Provided for Student Work

Chapter 5 Test

Name the base (and related unit) in SI.

1. length = _____   4. time = _____

2. mass (weight) = _____   5. volume = _____

3. temperature = _____

Write the correct abbreviations for the following:

6. milliliter _____   9. microgram _____

7. liter _____   10. kilogram _____

8. cubic centimeter _____   11. gram _____

How would you chart the following:

12. $\frac{1}{4}$ milliliter by intramuscular injection twice a day _____

13. three and one-half cubic centimeters in the morning _____

14. one-half gram at bedtime _____

15. twenty-five milligrams every 6 hours _____

16. three and two-tenths kilogram _____

17. one thousand milliliters by IV drip _____

18. fifteen milliliters as needed _____

Write the correct number.

19. Normal room temperature is about _____°C

20. Normal body temperature is about _____°C

21. Warm bath temperature is about _____°C

Convert each of the following to the unit requested:

22. 1000 ml = _____ ℓ 29. 5000 μg = _____ mg

23. 5 ml = _____ cc   30. 450 ml = _____ ℓ

24. 1.5 m = _____ cm   31. 975 mg = _____ g

25. 75 mg = _____ g   32. 20 kg = _____ g

26. 0.55g = _____ mg   33. 20 000 μg = _____ g

27. 0.45 ℓ = _____ cm^3 34. 3:00 P.M. = _____

28. 1250 mg = _____ g   35. 7:15 A.M. = _____

Complete the following:

36. 150 cc of H_2O weigh _____ g

37. 2.5 ℓ of H_2O weigh _____ kg

38. 0.036 kg is the weight of _____ cm^3 of water

39. Average weight of a newborn baby might be _____ kg.
    (3, 30, or 300)

40. Ordered: 25 mg prednisone
    Available: 10 mg tabs
    How many do you give? _____

41. Ordered: 250 mg of a medication
    Available: 125 mg tabs
    How many do you give? _____

42. If 3 ml of blood contains 2.5 g of hemoglobin, how much hemoglobin would you expect to find in 1.3 ml of blood? (round to tenths)

43. The English system uses fractions. The metric system uses _____.

Chapter 6

Converting Between the Apothecaries' and Metric Systems

This chapter explains how to convert between different systems of measurement. When you complete this chapter you should be able to:

a. Convert a measure from one system to a different system using proportions or the factor-label method.
b. Identify the appropriate conversion unit from the "Approximate Equivalents" table.
c. Convert temperature between Celsius and Fahrenheit.

6.1   Conversion Methods

A **conversion** or **equivalent** is a quantity in one system of measure that is equal to a quantity in another system of measure. Sometimes the medication on hand may not be labeled in the same system as that written on the physician's order sheet. Therefore, you may have to calculate an equivalent measure in another system. First, check a standard table of approximate equivalents (the conversion table). The printed cards for use with this text contain approximations. Many local hospitals will have their own conversion tables, and you may find that hospitals do not agree on all conversions. This text uses the conversions printed on the table, with the understanding that there will be some discrepancies at different hospitals. **This text is interested in the conversion process, rather than the exact conversion equivalents.** A 10% margin of error is considered acceptable by the Pharmacopoeia of the United States of America. For example, the conversion: 15 or 16 grains = 1 gram. One nurse may use 15 and another may use 16 in a conversion problem. Both are correct, since a 10% deviation is permitted when converting one system to another. This text will always choose the conversion unit that will require the simplest arithmetic. A more precise table of equivalents (conversion units) is presented in Appendix B.

For system-to-system conversions (called external conversions), use a proportion or the factor-label method. Recall that for conversions within a system (called internal conversions), you also use a proportion or the factor-label method, and within the metric system, you may use the metric conversion chart.

Proportion Conversion
On one side of the proportion, write the unit given to you in the numerator and the unit desired in the denominator. On the other side of the proportion, use the conversion from the card. Be sure the labels match on both sides of the proportion.

TO CONVERT UNITS USING A PROPORTION:

$$\frac{\text{Given amount}}{\text{Desired unit}} = \text{conversion equivalent as a fraction}$$

Factor-Label Conversion
Start with the amount given. Multiply this by a fraction with the desired unit in the numerator and the given unit in the denominator; then put the conversion amounts into this fraction using the conversion table. The old units will cancel and the desired unit will remain. Do the arithmetic as indicated.

TO CONVERT UNITS USING FACTOR-LABEL METHOD:

$$\text{Given amount} \times \frac{\text{Conversion unit Desired}}{\text{Conversion unit Given}} = \text{Desired amount}$$

Try working problems using both methods. After doing several problems, you will find that one of the methods will be easier for you to use and understand when doing external conversions.

Example: 56 grains = _____ grams

Before you begin, look up the conversion between grains and grams. The table shows: 16 grains = 1 gram

Using a proportion

$$\frac{56 \text{ grains}}{X \text{ grams}} = \frac{16 \text{ grains}}{1 \text{ gram}} \qquad \text{the conversion unit is on one side}$$

$$16 \, X = 56 \qquad \text{cross multiply}$$

$$X = 3.5 \text{ grams}$$

Using factor-label method

$$56 \text{ grains} \times \frac{1 \text{ gram}}{16 \text{ grains}} = \frac{56}{16} \text{ grams} = 3.5 \text{ grams}$$

Use an equal sign to express the answer, but remember that this conversion is approximate. Using 15 grains = 1 gram, the answer would be 3.7 grams.

Example: 20 ml = _____ tsp.

Look up the conversion between milliliters and teaspoons. The approximate conversion is: 5 ml = 1 tsp.

Using a proportion

$$\frac{20 \text{ ml}}{X \text{ tsp.}} = \frac{5 \text{ ml}}{1 \text{ tsp.}} \qquad \text{the conversion unit is on one side}$$

$$5X = 20$$

$$X = 4 \text{ tsp.}$$

Using factor-label method

$$20 \text{ ml} \times \frac{1 \text{ tsp.}}{5 \text{ ml}} = \frac{20}{5} \text{ tsp.} = 4 \text{ tsp.}$$

Problems to try. Answers to these problems appear at the end of 6.1 exercises.

a.   45 grains = _____ grams   c.   5 drams = _____ ml

b.   124 mg = _____ grains   d.   143 lbs. = _____ kg

6.1   Exercises

Use one of the conversion methods to convert each of the following to the desired unit.

1. 3 g = _____ gr.   2. $4\frac{1}{2}$ oz. = _____ cc

3. 255 mg = _____ gr.   4. 20 dr. = _____ ml

5. 50 mg = _____ g   6. 0.6 ℓ = _____ ml

7. 15 gr. = _____ mg   8. 150 ml = _____ oz.

9. 90 gr. = _____ g   10. 60 ♏$_x$ = _____ ml

11. 12 ml = _____ dr.   12. 150 lbs. = _____ kg

13. 7.5 gr. = _____ g   14. 15 ml = _____ tsp.

15. 3 tsp. = _____ ml   16. 250 ml = _____ pt.

Do the following conversions using the given unit from charted symbols, and writing the answer in charted symbols. Note: some of these are "internal" conversions.

17. ℥v = _____ g   18. f℈ii = _____ ♏$_x$

19. gr. x = _____ g   20. ℥iiss = _____ cc

21. 10 ml = ℥ _____

22. 3 Tbsp. = dr. _____

23. ♏ 45 = _____ ml

24. 8 ml = ♏ _____

25. $\frac{1}{2}$ pt. = _____ ml

26. gr. xxx = _____ g

Answers to Problems to try.

a. 3 g   b. 2 gr.   c. 20 ml   d. 65 kg

_____

Space Provided for Student Work

_____

6.2   Word Problems

The following word problems require a preliminary conversion step before finding the amount to give the patient. In general, **convert the doctor's order to agree with the unit in which the medication is dispensed.**

Remember: Total medication = Amount per tabet × Number of Tablets

Number of tablets = Total medication ÷ Amount per tablet

Read the problem until you understand what is given and what must be found. When you get the answer, go back and read the problem to see if your answer makes sense.

Example: Ordered: 2 g of a medication
Available: tablets containing 15 grains each.
Give _____ tablets.

The doctor's orders should first be converted to agree with the unit in which the medication is dispensed. Look up the conversion unit between grams and grains. The conversion is: 15 or 16 grains = 1 gram

Using a proportion to convert the doctor's order:

$$\frac{2 \text{ g}}{X \text{ grains}} = \frac{1 \text{ g}}{15 \text{ gr.}} \quad \text{cross multiplying}$$

$$1 X = 2(15) \qquad X = 30 \text{ grains}$$

Using factor-label method to convert the doctor's order:

$$2 \text{ g} \times \frac{15 \text{ gr.}}{1 \text{ g}} = 30 \text{ gr. so the doctor ordered 2 g} = 30 \text{ grains}$$

After converting the doctor's order to agree with the label unit, solve the word problem.

$$30 \text{ gr.} \div 15 \text{ gr.} = \frac{30}{15} = 2 \text{ tabs} \qquad \text{Give the patient 2 tablets.}$$

Example: A doctor orders 15 grains of medication to be divided into three doses. It is available in 200 mg tablets. How many tablets should you give each dose? (Realistically, doctors do not order medication in grains. However, the intent here is to examine the conversion process.)

Since the medication is divided into three doses, divide 15 grains in three doses of 5 grains each before starting the problem. Your final answer will be the divided dosage.

Next, convert the doctor's order to agree with the milligram unit on the label. The conversion unit is: 1 gr. = 60 mg

Using a proportion

$$\frac{5 \text{ gr.}}{X \text{ mg}} = \frac{1 \text{ gr.}}{60 \text{ mg}}$$

$$1 X = 5(6) \qquad X = 300 \text{ mg}$$

Using factor-label method

$$5 \text{ gr.} \times \frac{60 \text{ mg}}{1 \text{ gr.}} = 300 \text{ mg}$$

Now calculate the amount to give the patient:

$$300 \text{ mg} \div 200 \text{ mg} = 1\frac{1}{2} \text{ tablets}$$

Example: A patient weighs 130 pounds. If you are to give 5 mg for every kg of body weight, how much would you give this patient?

First, convert the patient's weight to kilograms.

Using a proportion

$$\frac{130 \text{ lb.}}{X \text{ kg}} = \frac{2.2 \text{ lb.}}{1 \text{ kg}}$$

$$2.2 X = 130$$

$$X = \frac{130}{2.2} = 59 \text{ kg}$$

Using factor-label method

$$130 \text{ lb.} \times \frac{1 \text{ kg}}{2.2 \text{ lb.}} = 59 \text{ kg}$$

Now solve the problem:

$$59 \text{ kg} \times \frac{5 \text{ mg}}{1 \text{ kg}} = 295 \text{ mg} \qquad \text{This patient should receive 295 mg.}$$

6.2   *Exercises*

1. A doctor orders 5 gr. of medication. The medication is available in 100 mg tablets. How many tablets should you give? If the medication came in 150 mg tablets, how many should you give?

2. A doctor orders $1\frac{1}{2}$ grains. The label on the medication reads: "each tablet contains 93 milligrams." How many tablets should you give?

3. Ordered: 18 grains to be divided into 6 doses. You have on hand capsules containing 0.1 gram each. How many capsules will you give per dose?

4. Ordered: gr. $1\frac{7}{8}$
    On hand: tablets containing 120 mg each.
    Give _____ tablets.

5. Ordered: gr. iiss
    Available: 75 mg tablets
    Give _____ tablets.

6. An infant is to be given 4 oz. of formula every four hours. The formula comes in 200 ml cans. How many cans should you order for a three-day supply?

7. Ordered: gr. iv q.4h.
    Available: tablets labeled 125 mg each.
    Give _____ tablets.

8. The atropine sulfate label reads 0.4 mg per ml. Calculate the number of milliliters to give if the doctor's order requires gr. $\frac{1}{150}$ atropine sulfate.

9. A patient weighs 154 pounds. What is the patient's weight in kilograms? If you are to give 5 mg for every kg of body weight, how many mg would you give the patient?

10. Ordered: ℥ ̄iss q.i.d. antacid. How many days would a 360 ml bottle last?

11. An aspirin tablet contains 5 grains. If you give 2 tablets (10 grain) how many milligrams have you given?

12. A 12-year-old child with acute asthma weights 71 lbs. You are to give 6 mg of aminophylline IV over a 20-minute period for every kg of body weight. How many milligrams do you give?

13. You must prepare solution for 6 compresses. Each require 250 ml. How many quarts do you prepare?

14. A doctor orders 60 ℳ$_x$ per dose. You have on hand a 32 ml bottle. How many doses can you get out of the bottle?

15. A doctor orders gr. $\frac{1}{5}$ daily to be given in divided doses b.i.d. The medication is available in 2 mg tablets. How many do you give per dose?

16. If the doctor prescribes 10 ml, how many teaspoons would you tell the patient to take at home?

17. If the doctor prescribes ℨ̄ss, how many teaspoons would you tell the patient to take at home?

18. You must prepare a solution for 12 irrigations during the day. Each one requires ℨ̄ xvi of solution. How many liters total are needed for one day?

19. A patient weighs 175 pounds. If you are to give 7 mg for every kg of body weight, how many mg should you give this patient?

20. A patient weighs 220 pounds. If you are to give 5 mg for every kg of body weight, how many mg should you give this patient?

Space Provided for Student Work

6.3   Temperature Conversion

There are special formulas to use for temperature conversion. Round temperature conversions to the tenths place.

TO CONVERT BETWEEN CELSIUS AND FAHRENHEIT:

$$C = \frac{5}{9}(F - 32) \quad \text{and} \quad F = \frac{9}{5}C + 32$$

Example: $40°C =$ _____ $°F$

Using the second formula:

$$F = \frac{9}{5}(4) + 32 = 72 + 32 = 104° \ F$$

Notice that the fraction $\frac{9}{5}$ is multiplied by 40 **before** adding 32.

Example: $113°F =$ _____ $°C$

Using the first formula:

$$C = \frac{5}{9}(113 - 32) = \frac{5}{9}(81) = 45°C$$

Notice that 32 is first subtracted from the Fahrenheit temperature, and then the result is multiplied by the fraction $\frac{5}{9}$.

The fractions $\frac{5}{9}$ and $\frac{9}{5}$ can be changed to decimal equivalents and substituted into the temperature formulas:

$$C = 0.556 \ (F - 32) \quad \text{and} \quad F = 1.8C + 32$$

Calculations are done in the same order as in the examples above, using the decimals instead of the fractions. Answers should be rounded to the nearest tenth of a degree.

Example: $40°C = $ _____ $°F$

Using the second formula:

$F = (1.8 \times 40) + 32 = 72 + 32 = 104°F$

Example: $113°\ F = $ _____ $°C$

Using the first formula:

$C = 0.556(113 - 32) = 0.556(81) = 45°C$

6.3   Exercises

Convert the following to the required unit:

1. $106°F = $ _____ $°C$ 2. $45°C = $ _____ $°F$

3. $14°C = $ _____ $°F$ 4. $88°F = $ _____ $°C$

5. $39.5°C = $ _____ $°F$ 6. $98.6°F = $ _____ $°C$

7. $72°F = $ _____ $°C$ 8. $20°C = $ _____ $°F$

9. $43°C = $ _____ $°F$ 10. $103°F = $ _____ $°C$

11. $32°\ F = $ _____ $°C$ 12. $100.2°F = $ _____ $°C$

13. The USP defines a refrigerator as a place that stores medications between 2 and 8 degrees Celsius. What is the equivalent range in degrees Fahrenheit?

Chapter 6 Test

Do the following conversions, writing the answers in charted symbols.

1. 0.5 ℓ = f ℥ _____

2. f ℥ īss= _____ ml

3. lb. $\frac{1}{4}$ = _____ g

4. qt. iii = _____ ℓ

5. ♏ xv = _____ ml

6. ℥ īi = _____ g

Circle the **smaller** unit.

7. ℥ ī   or   6 cc

8. 60 ml   or   f ℥ ī

9. ℥ īi   or   6 g

10. gr. 45   or   5 g

11. 60 kg   or   135 lb.

Solve the following word problems.

12. Atropine gr. $\frac{1}{150}$ is a standard pre-operative dose. How many mg is the patient receiving?

13. Ordered: 5cc q.6h. for 6 days. How many total ounces is this?

14. A patient is to receive $\frac{1}{2}$ tsp. q.6h. You have a 50 ml bottle on hand. How many doses will you get out of the bottle? How many days will the bottle last?

15. Ordered: NEMBUTAL® gr. $\overline{\text{iss}}$
    On hand: capsules labeled 50 mg each
    Give _____ capsules.

16. Ordered: DILANTIN® gr. v
    On hand: capsules labeled 100 mg each
    Give _____ capsules.

17. Ordered: morphine gr. ss q.4h. p.r.n.
    On hand: 15 mg tablets
    Give _____ tablets per dose.

18. Ordered: nitroglycerin gr. $\frac{1}{150}$ p.r.n.
    On hand: 0.4 mg tablets
    Give _____ tablets per dose.

19. The dosage of a medication is 5 mg per kilogram of body weight. A child weighs 17.6 pounds. How many kg does the child weigh? How many milligrams should you give this child?

20. An infant receives 6 oz. of formula every four hours. How many 500 ml cans are needed for a four-day supply?

21. If a patient receives one-half of a 5-grain tablet every 8 hours, how many total milligrams has he received after 2 days?

22. Ordered: DILANTIN® gr. $\overline{\text{iiss}}$
    Available: 50 mg tablets
    Give _____ tablets.

23. Convert: 39°C = _____°F

24. Convert: 103°F = _____°C

Chapter 7

Dosages and Solutions

This chapter explains label information and dosage calculations. When you complete this chapter you should be able to:

a. Interpret medication strengths from the label.
b. Calculate patient dosage (using one of four formulas) from either prepared solutions or reconstituted solutions.
c. Calculate patient dosage from medications in powdered form that must be diluted prior to administration.
d. Date and label vials after a powdered medication has been diluted.
e. Find the amount of medication in a given solution.
f. Calculate amount of concentrated solution and diluent needed for dilution to a desired strength.
g. Calculate pediatric dosages by child's body weight, when medications are labeled in mg/kg/day or mg/lb./day.
h. Calculate patient dosage using a nomogram.

7.1   Interpreting Labels

Nurses administer medication orally (P.O.), intramuscularly (IM), subcutaneously (SC or SQ), or through IV fluids from a prepared solution (stock solution). The strength of the solution is stated on the label.

163

Solution strengths are usually labeled in one of the following ways:

Label Information	Meaning
a. 25 mg/ml	This ratio tells the amount of medication in each ml of solution.
b. 1:4	Ratios written this way always mean grams per milliliter. This solution contains 1 gram of medication in every 4 ml of solution.
c. 30%	Percentages describe the amount of medication (in grams) in every 100 ml of solution. This solution contains 30 grams of medication in every 100 ml.
d. 40 mg = 2 cc	This equation tells the amount of medication in the given volume.
e. U-100	Certain solutions list units per ml. This solution contains 100 units per ml.
f. 20 mEq/ml	This ratio tells the number of milli-equivalents per milliliter of solution.

Example: What does 25% strength mean?

Answer: 25% means 25 grams of medication in every 100 ml of solution

---

7.1   Exercises

Interpret this label information.

1.   2:5   _____

2.   15%   _____

3.   U-100   _____

4.   20 mg/cc   _____

5.   300 mg = 10 ml   _____

6. 1:1000 _____

7. 60 mg/ml _____

8. 20% _____

9. 20 mg = 3 ml _____

10. 1:10 _____

Interpret the medication strength from these labels.

11.

```
┌─────────────────────────────────────────┐
│              2 ml vial                    │
│         CLEOCIN® PHOSPHATE                │
│            sterile solution               │
│   clindamycin phosphate injection, USP    │
│                300 mg                     │
└─────────────────────────────────────────┘
```

12.

```
┌─────────────────────────────────────────┐
│  10 dosette vials-each contains 1 ml      │
│             MEPERIDINE                    │
│           HCL injection USP               │
│                                           │
│               50 mg/ml                    │
└─────────────────────────────────────────┘
```

13.

```
┌─────────────────────────────────────────┐
│           DELIVERS 15 ml                  │
│             POTASSIUM                     │
│             CHLORIDE                      │
│          20 mEq per 15 ml                 │
└─────────────────────────────────────────┘
```

14.

```
┌─────────────────────────────────────────┐
│               16 fl oz                    │
│          ILOSONE LIQUID®                  │
│         erythromycin estolate             │
│        oral suspension, USP               │
│           250 mg per 5 ml                 │
└─────────────────────────────────────────┘
```

16.

```
┌─────────────────────────────────────────┐
│            120 ml vial                    │
│             VISTARIL®                     │
│        hydroxyzine pamoate                │
│           oral suspension                 │
│             25 mg/5 ml                    │
└─────────────────────────────────────────┘
```

17.

```
┌─────────────────────────────────────────┐
│        200 ml (when mixed)                │
│              KEFLEX®                      │
│  cephalexin for oral suspension, USP      │
│                                           │
│           125 mg per 5 ml                 │
└─────────────────────────────────────────┘
```

7.2   Dosage Calculations for Prepared Solutions

There are four acceptable ways of calculating solution dosages—the amount (dosage) to give to the patient. All are mathematically equivalent.

1. **Dosage Formula**

   This formula is unique to this book. It is most closely related to the factor-label method for conversions between measurement systems. The value of this formula is that the labels (unit of measure) act as a double check for the answer if they cancel correctly. The answer is the exact volume (or number of tablets) to give to the patient.

Doctor orders ÷ label information = patient dosage

---

2. **DQA Proportion**

   The letters in this formula represent: D = "desired"; Q = "quantity"; A = "available". The bottom of the proportion (the denominators) correspond to the label information. The patient's dosage is called the "quantity to give".

$$\frac{\textbf{Desired amount}}{\textbf{Available amount}} = \frac{\textbf{Quantity to give}}{\textbf{Quantity on hand}}$$

---

3. **DHQ Formula**

   The letters in this formula represent: D = "desired" or the amount ordered; H = "have" or the amount of medication in the solution; Q = "quantity" or the volume of the solution; and X = "unknown" or amount to give patient. (Note: H and Q are label information)

$$\frac{\textbf{D}}{\textbf{H}} \times \textbf{Q} = \textbf{X} \quad \textit{means} \quad \frac{\textbf{desired}}{\textbf{have}} \times \textbf{quantity} = \textbf{unknown}$$

---

4. **Label Proportion**

One side of this proportion is the exact information from the medication label. The other side contains the doctor's order and the patient's dosage (amount to give).

$$\frac{\text{Doctor Orders}}{\text{Amount to give}} = \frac{\text{Medication weight}}{\text{Solution volume}}$$

Try working problems using all four formulas. After doing several problems, you may select one of the formulas that is easier for you to understand and use in calculating dosages.

Example: The doctor orders 60 mg of a medication. The medication comes in a solution labeled 1:5. How many ml of solution will you administer?

Note: The strength 1:5 means there is 1 gram of medication in every 5 ml of solution. You will first need to convert 1 gram into 1000 mg to agree with the milligram unit in the doctor's orders.

1. Using the **Dosage Formula**

$$60 \text{ mg} \div \frac{1 \text{ g}}{5 \text{ ml}} = 60 \text{ mg} \times \frac{5 \text{ ml}}{1000 \text{ mg}} = \frac{300 \text{ ml}}{1000} = 0.3 \text{ ml}$$

2. Using the **DQA Proportion**

$$\frac{60 \text{ mg}}{1 \text{ g}} = \frac{X \text{ ml}}{5 \text{ ml}} \quad \text{or} \quad \frac{60 \text{ mg}}{1000 \text{ mg}} = \frac{X \text{ ml}}{5 \text{ ml}}$$

$$1000 \text{ X} = 300 \qquad X = \frac{300}{1000} = 0.3 \text{ ml}$$

3. Using the **DHQ Formula**

$$\frac{60 \text{ mg}}{1 \text{ g}} \times 5 \text{ ml} = \frac{60 \text{ mg}}{1000 \text{ mg}} \times 5 \text{ ml} = \frac{300}{1000} = 0.3 \text{ ml}$$

4. Using the **Label Proportion**

$$\frac{60 \text{ mg}}{X \text{ ml}} = \frac{1 \text{ g}}{5 \text{ ml}} \quad \text{or} \quad \frac{60 \text{ mg}}{X \text{ ml}} = \frac{1000 \text{ mg}}{5 \text{ ml}}$$

$$1000 \text{ X} = 300 \qquad X = \frac{300}{1000} = 0.3 \text{ ml}$$

Using any of the four formulas, the correct answer is: 60 mg = 0.3 ml

Example: The doctor orders 50 mg. The medication comes in a 10% solution. How many milliliters will you give to the patient?

Note: The label 10% means there are 10 grams of medication in every 100 ml of solution. Convert 10 grams to 10,000 mg to agree with the milligram unit in the doctor's orders.

1. Using the **Dosage Formula**

$$50 \text{ mg} \div \frac{10 \text{ g}}{100 \text{ ml}} = 50 \text{ mg} \times \frac{100 \text{ ml}}{10000 \text{ mg}} = 0.5 \text{ ml}$$

2. Using the **DQA Proportion**

$$\frac{50 \text{ mg}}{10 \text{ g}} = \frac{X \text{ ml}}{100 \text{ ml}} \quad \text{or} \quad \frac{50 \text{ mg}}{10000 \text{ mg}} = \frac{X \text{ m}}{100 \text{ ml}}$$

$$10000 \text{ X} = 5000 \qquad X = \frac{5000}{10000} = 0.5 \text{ ml}$$

3. Using the **DHQ Formula**

$$\frac{50 \text{ mg}}{10 \text{ g}} \times 100 \text{ ml} = \frac{50 \text{ mg}}{10000 \text{ mg}} \times 100 \text{ ml} = 0.5 \text{ ml}$$

4. Using the **Label Proportion**

$$\frac{50 \text{ mg}}{X \text{ ml}} = \frac{10 \text{ g}}{100 \text{ ml}} \quad \text{or} \quad \frac{50 \text{ mg}}{X \text{ ml}} = \frac{10000 \text{ mg}}{100 \text{ ml}}$$

$$10000 \text{ X} = 5000$$

$$X = 0.5 \text{ ml}$$

The answer is: 50 mg = 0.5 ml

Example: The doctor orders gr. vi P.O. q.d. The medication comes in a solution strength of 25 mg/cc. How many cc's do you give?

Note: The doctor has ordered in the apothecaries' system. First convert this order to the metric equivalent before using one of the four dosage calculation formulas.

$$\text{Conversion: 6 grains} \times \frac{60 \text{ mg}}{1 \text{ grain}} = 360 \text{ mg}$$

1. Using the **Dosage Formula**

    $$360 \text{ mg} \div \frac{25 \text{ mg}}{1 \text{ cc}} = 360 \text{ mg} \times \frac{1 \text{ cc}}{25 \text{ mg}} = 14 \text{ cc}$$

2. Using the **DQA Proportion**

    $$\frac{360 \text{ mg}}{25 \text{ mg}} = \frac{X \text{ cc}}{1 \text{ cc}}$$

    $$25 X = 360$$

    $$X = 14 \text{ cc}$$

3. Using the **DHQ Formula**

    $$\frac{360 \text{ mg}}{25 \text{ mg}} \times 1 \text{ cc} = 14 \text{ cc}$$

4. Using the **Label Proportion**

    $$\frac{360 \text{ mg}}{X \text{ cc}} = \frac{25 \text{ mg}}{1 \text{ cc}}$$

    $$25 X = 360$$

    $$X = 14 \text{ cc}$$

The amount calculated to give the patient is approximately 14 cc. Although the conversion from apothecaries' to metric was approximate (1 gr. = 60–65 mg), and answers may vary slightly, write: 6 grains = 14 cc.

Problems to try. Answers to these problems appear at the end of 7.2 exercises.

Using one or more of the dosage calculation formulas, calculate the dosage to give to the patient.

a. Ordered: 15 mg IM q.a.m.
    Label info: 20 mg/ml
    Patient dosage: _____

b. Ordered: 25 mg IM b.i.d.
    Label info: 1:4 strength solution
    Patient dosage: _____

c. Ordered: 50 mg P.O. q.p.m.
    Label: 25 mg = 2 ml
    Patient dosage: _____

Units

Insulin, heparin, some penicillin, and ACTH are manufactured in units rather than milligrams. These medications are listed as having a stated number of USP units. The USP designation refers to the fact that the composition of the unit conforms to specifications laid down by the United States Pharmacopoeia, the official drug publication of the US government. The doctor will usually prescribe the dosage in units. U-100 is the standard form for insulin, meaning 100 units per milliliter. Previously, insulin was dispersed in U-40 and U-80 as well as U-100. In April 1980, U-40 and U-80 were phased out.

Example: Give 30 units of U-100.

If you are told to give 30 units of U-100 **from an insulin syringe**, draw to the 30 unit mark and administer. Insulin syringes are marked in units.

If you are told to give 30 units of U-100 **from a syringe graduated in milliliters (or cc's)**, use one of the dosage calculation formulas to determine how many milliliters to give to the patient.

1. Using the **Dosage Formula**

$$30 \text{ U} \div \frac{100 \text{ U}}{1 \text{ ml}} = 30 \text{ U} \times \frac{1 \text{ ml}}{100 \text{ U}} = \frac{30 \text{ U}}{100 \text{ U}} = 0.3 \text{ ml}$$

2. Using the **DQA Proportion**

$$\frac{30 \text{ U}}{100 \text{ U}} = \frac{X \text{ ml}}{1 \text{ ml}}$$

$$100 \text{ X} = 30$$

$$X = 0.3 \text{ ml}$$

3. Using the **DHQ Formula**

$$\frac{30 \text{ U}}{100 \text{ U}} \times 1 \text{ ml} = 0.3 \text{ ml}$$

4. Using the **Label Proportion**

$$\frac{30 \text{ units}}{X \text{ ml}} = \frac{100 \text{ units}}{1 \text{ ml}}$$

$$100 \, X = 30$$

$$X = \frac{30}{100} = 0.3 \text{ ml}$$

Answer: draw the syringe to the 0.3 cc mark and administer.

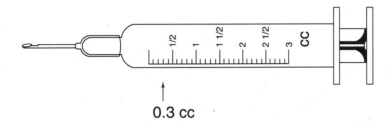

0.3 cc

Problems to try. Answers to these problems appear at the end of 7.2 exercises.

d. How many ml of insulin are needed to give 150 units of U-100?

e. How many ml of insulin are needed to give 80 units of U-100?

f. How many ml of insulin are needed to give 60 units of U-100?

Milliequivalents
Some medications are measured in amounts called milliequivalents (mEq). When mEq medications are added to an IV, they are usually added to 1 liter (1000 ml) of IV fluid. Milliequivalent weight is 1/1000 of an equivalent weight. Milliequivalent is used so the relatively small quantities found in medicine can be expressed in whole numbers. The term "154 milliequivalents of sodium per liter" (154 mEq/ℓ) means there are 154 thousandths of an equivalent weight of sodium in one liter of normal saline solution. To find the mEq volume to give the patient (either added to the IV fluid or given orally), use one of the dosage calculation formulas.

Example: Ordered: 36 mEq to IV fluids
              Medication label: 3 mEq/ml
              How many ml will you add to the IV fluids?

1. **Dosage Formula**

$$36 \text{ mEq} \div \frac{3 \text{ mEq}}{1 \text{ ml}} = 36 \text{ mEq} \times \frac{1 \text{ ml}}{3 \text{ mEq}} = 12 \text{ ml}$$

2. **DQA Proportion**

$$\frac{36 \text{ mEq}}{3 \text{ mEq}} = \frac{X \text{ ml}}{1 \text{ ml}}$$

$$3X = 36$$

$$X = 12 \text{ ml}$$

3. **DHQ Formula**

$$\frac{36 \text{ mEq}}{3 \text{ mEq}} \times 1 \text{ ml} = 12 \text{ ml}$$

4. **Label Proportion**

$$\frac{36 \text{ mEq}}{X \text{ ml}} = \frac{3 \text{ mEq}}{1 \text{ ml}}$$

$$3X = 36$$

$$X = 12 \text{ ml}$$

Answer: add 12 ml to the IV fluids

Problems to try. Answers to these problems appear at the end of 7.2 exercises.

g. Ordered: 6 mEq medication in 1000 ml IV fluid
   Medication label: 1.5 mEq/ml
   How many ml will you add to the IV fluid? _____

h. Ordered: 3 mEq of a medication
   Available: 1.5 mEq/ml
   How many ml will you administer? _____

When milliequivalent medication is given orally, it is usually administered in divided dosages. To find the volume to give the patient, use one of the dosage calculation formulas.

Example: Ordered: 15 mEq P.O. t.i.d.
                  Label info: 30 mEq = 14 ml
                  How many ml per dose?   _____

1. **Dosage Formula**

$$15 \text{ mEq} \div \frac{30 \text{ mEq}}{14 \text{ ml}} = 15 \text{ mEq} \times \frac{14 \text{ ml}}{30 \text{ mEq}} = \frac{210 \text{ ml}}{30} = 7 \text{ ml}$$

2. **DQA Proportion**

$$\frac{15 \text{ mEq}}{30 \text{ mEq}} = \frac{X \text{ ml}}{14 \text{ ml}}$$

$$30 X = 15(14) = 210$$

$$X = \frac{210}{30} = 7 \text{ ml}$$

3. **DHQ Formula**

$$\frac{15 \text{ mEq}}{30 \text{ mEq}} \times 14 \text{ ml} = 7 \text{ ml}$$

4. **Label Proportion**

$$\frac{15 \text{ mEq}}{X \text{ ml}} = \frac{30 \text{ mEq}}{14 \text{ ml}}$$

$$30 X = 210$$

$$X = 7 \text{ ml}$$

Give 7 ml orally per dose, 3 times a day.

Problems to try. Answers to these problems appear at the end of 7.2 exercises.

i. Ordered: 80 mEq P.O. q.6h.
   Label info: 20 mEq = 5 ml
   How many ml do you give per dose?   _____

j. Ordered: 8.5 mEq magnesium sulfate
   Label info: magnesium sulfate 81.2 mEq/100 ml
   How many ml do you give?   _____

Geriatric Patients

The elderly patient presents special needs and problems related to medication administration. Lower dosages of medication are frequently needed due to the numerous factors that affect their body's ability to process and assimilate medication. These may include:

- advancing age
- decreased metabolism
- multiple medications
- multiple diagnosis
- poor nutritional status
- deteriorating mental condition

Because of the problems, the normal dosage of medication may need to be altered by the doctor.

7.2   Exercises

Calculate the patient dosage (volume) needed to fill the doctor's orders.

1. Ordered: 25 mg IM t.i.d.
   Label into: solution strength 50 mg per ml
   Patient dosage: _____

2. Ordered: 15 mg IM q.a.m.
   Label: 20 mg/ml
   Patient dosage: _____

3. Ordered: 50 mg P.O.
   Label: 25 mg = 2 ml
   Patient dosage: _____

4. Ordered: 60 U of U-100 insulin
   Calculate how much to give from a syringe marked in cc's: _____

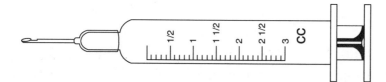

5. Ordered: 6 mEq potassium chloride (oral)
    Label: 40 mEq/30 ml
    Patient dosage: _____

6. Ordered: 30 mEq potassium added to IV solution
    Label: 20 mEq = 5 ml

    Patient dosage: _____

7. Ordered: 0.15 mg SC
    Label:

    ```
    20 ml vial
    ATROPINE SULFATE
    injection, USP
    0.4 mg (1/150 gr.) per ml
    ```

    Patient dosage: _____

8. Ordered: erythromycin 250 mg P.O. q.6h.
    Label:

    ```
    100 ml vial
    ILOSONE LIQUID®
    erythromycin estolate
    oral suspension, USP
    250 mg per 5 ml
    ```

    Patient dosage: _____

9. Ordered: erythromycin 150 mg P.O. q.6h.
    Label:

    ```
    100 ml vial
    ILOSONE LIQUID®
    erythromycin estolate
    oral suspension, USP
    250 mg per 5 ml
    ```

    Patient dosage: _____

10.   Ordered: DEMEROL® (meperidine hydrochloride) 75 mg
       Available: vial labeled 1 ml = 25 mg
       How many ml do you give?   _____

11.   Ordered: KEFLEX® 75 mg P.O. q.6h.
       Label:

200 ml (when mixed) **KEFLEX®** *cephalexin for oral suspension, USP* 125 mg per 5 ml

       Patient dosage: _____

12.   Ordered: VISTARIL® 50 mg P.O. q.i.d.
       Label:

120 ml vial **VISTARIL®** hydroxyzine pamoate oral suspension 25 mg / 5 ml

       Patient dosage: _____

13.   Ordered: morphine sulfate gr. $\frac{1}{4}$
       Label:

20 dosette vials—each contains 1 ml **MORPHINE SULFATE** INJECTION, USP 15 mg/ml

       Patient dosage: _____

14.   Ordered: sodium heparin 2000 U SQ
       Available: 5 ml vial labeled 10 000 U/ml
       How many ml do you administer?   _____

15. Ordered: sodium heparin 500 U SQ
     Available: 10 ml vial labeled 1 ml = 1000 U
     How many ml do you administer? _____

16. Ordered: DEMEROL® (meperidine hydrochloride) 75 mg
     Available: vial labeled 1 ml = 50 mg
     How many ml do you give? _____

17. Ordered: VALIUM® (diazepam) 5 mg IM
     Available: vial labeled 2 ml = 10 mg
     How many ml do you administer? _____

18. Ordered: medication 175 000 U b.i.d.
     Label: medication 350 000 U/ml. Keep refrigerated. Stable 7 days.
     How many ml do you give per dose? _____

19. Ordered: procaine hydrochloride 375 mg
     Label: procaine hydrochloride 15% solution
     How many ml do you give? _____

20. Ordered: epinephrine 10 μg per kg body weight
     Patient weight: 35 kg
     Available: 1:1000 solution
     How many ml do you give? _____

21. Ordered: gr. $\frac{1}{30}$
     Label: 0.1% solution
     How many ml do you give? _____

22. Ordered: gr. $\frac{1}{200}$
     Label: 0.05% solution
     How many ml do you give? _____

23. Ordered: VISTARIL® (hydroxyzine pamoate) 0.1 g
     Label: 100 mg/2 ml
     How many ml do you give? _____

24. What is the percent strength of 1 ℥ of solution containing 5 g of solute?

25. Ordered: Children's Tylenol 8 mg   q.4h.   p.r.n. for temperature over
                     101°F.
     Available: Children's Tylenol solution 60 mg = 0.6 ml
     How many ml do you give? _____

26. Ordered: ampicillin 150 mg IM
     Available: vial containing 500 mg/ml
     How many ml do you administer? _____

Answers to Problems to try.

a. 0.75 ml   b. 0.1 ml   c. 4 ml   d. 1.5 ml   e. 0.8 ml   f. 0.6 ml

g. 4 ml   h. 2 ml   i. 20 ml   j. 10.5 ml

Space Provided for Student Work

7.3   Dosage Calculations from Medications In Powdered Form

Many medications, such as antibiotics, are unstable when stored in solution, and therefore are packed in powder or granular form in a vial. These medications must be dissolved before use by adding the sterile liquid to form a solution that will increase in volume. For example, if you need a total of 10 ml, you may only add 8.5 ml to form the final amount of 10 ml. The powder takes up the remaining volume.

Read the literature packaged with the medication for instructions regarding the type and amount of diluent to be added. The label on the medication will tell how much sterile liquid to add and the final volume to have in the vial. If more than one dose is to be given from a vial, **write the date and time of preparation directly on the vial, your initials, and the strength of the solution** if it is not already indicated on the label.

You will be told:

    a. The doctor's orders (charted amount)
    b. Label information

You will need to calculate:

    c. How much to give per dose (in ml or cc)
    d. How often to give it
    e. How to relabel the vial if it is multidose

When calculating how much to give per dose, use one of the dosage calculation formulas. Consistently use the formula you understand the best.

Many hospitals will require the nurse to put the patient's name on the multidose vial along with the patient dosage and time of preparation. This text does not require the patient name as part of the answer in the problems requiring relabeling.

Example: Ordered: 1.0 g IM q.6h.
                  Label reads: 4 g of medication—inject 5.7 ml sterile water to yield
                               8 ml of solution. Stable 24 hours at room temp.
                  How much do you give and how often? _____

Note: Before beginning the calculations, realize that the strength of the medication now in solution is 4 g in 8 ml. **Use medication strength in dosage calculations.**

1. **Dosage Formula**

$$1.0 \text{ g} \div \frac{4 \text{ g}}{8 \text{ ml}} = 1.0 \text{ g} \times \frac{8 \text{ ml}}{4 \text{ g}} = \frac{8}{4} \text{ ml} = 2 \text{ ml}$$

2. **DQA Proportion**

$$\frac{1 \text{ g}}{4 \text{ g}} = \frac{X \text{ ml}}{8 \text{ ml}}$$

$$4 \, X = 8$$

$$X = 2 \text{ ml}$$

3. **DHQ Formula**

$$\frac{1 \text{ g}}{4 \text{ g}} \times 8 \text{ ml} = \frac{8}{4} \text{ ml} = 2 \text{ ml}$$

4. **Label Proportion**

$$\frac{1 \text{ g}}{X \text{ ml}} = \frac{4 \text{ g}}{8 \text{ ml}}$$

$$4X = 8$$

$$X = 2 \text{ ml}$$

The amount to give the patient is 2 ml. The complete answer should read:

Give 2 ml IM every 6 hours.
Relabel the vial 1.0 g = 2 ml, with the date and time of preparation, and your initials.

Example: Ordered: 250 mg IM q.i.d.
Label information: 500 mg medication—inject 1.2 ml SW to yield 2 ml solution. Must be used within one hour.

How much do you give and how often?

Note: Before beginning the calculations, first determine that the medication strength is 500 g in 2 ml, or 250 mg per ml. Use medication strength in dosage calculations.

1. **Dosage Formula**

$$250 \text{ mg} \div \frac{500 \text{ mg}}{2 \text{ ml}} = 250 \text{ mg} \times \frac{2 \text{ ml}}{500 \text{ mg}} = \frac{500}{500} \text{ ml} = 1 \text{ ml}$$

2. **DQA Proportion**

$$\frac{250 \text{ mg}}{500 \text{ mg}} = \frac{X \text{ ml}}{2 \text{ ml}}$$

$$500 \text{ X} = 2(250)$$

$$X = \frac{500}{500} = 1 \text{ ml}$$

3. **DHQ Formula**

$$\frac{250 \text{ mg}}{500 \text{ mg}} \times 2 \text{ ml} = \frac{500}{500} \text{ ml} = 1 \text{ ml}$$

4. **Label Proportion**

$$\frac{250 \text{ mg}}{X \text{ ml}} = \frac{500 \text{ mg}}{2 \text{ ml}}$$

$$500 \text{ X} = 2(250)$$

$$X = \frac{500}{500} = 1 \text{ ml}$$

Answer: Give 1 ml IM four times a day. Discard vial after each injection, since this vial is not multidose and the solution is unstable.

Problems to try. Answers to these problems appear at the end of 7.3 exercises.

a. Ordered: 750 mg IM q.d. at 1000 hours (10 a.m.)
   Label information: 1.0 g medication—inject 1.5 ml sterile water to yield 2 ml
                                of solution. Stable for 6 hours.
   How much do you give and how often?   _____

b. Ordered: 250 mg   IM   t.i.d.
   Label information: 1.0 g medication—inject 1.7 ml sterile water to yield 2 ml
                                solution. Keep refrigerated. Stable for 3 days.
   How much do you give and how often?   _____

Choice of Strength Vials

Occasionally, the label may specify the amount the sterile liquid to add for various strengths of medication. In order to control the total volume of solution that results in reconstitution, the manufacturers provide specific dosages per specific amounts of solution. In this situation, the easiest arithmetic implies you should choose the strength closest to, but not exceeding, the ordered amount of medication, and then calculate the dosage using medication strength. If given IM, the least painful to the patient is the smallest amount; however, to avoid too heavy a concentration, try to choose a strength that will allow you to administer between 1 and 2 ml. This will usually be the strength closest to, but not exceeding, the ordered amount.

Example: Ordered: 750 000 Units penicillin G

Label info: The package insert of penicillin G 5 000 000 Units provides the following information:

Volume of Diluent	Concentration of Solution
3.2 ml	1 000 000 Units/ml
8.2 ml	500 000 Units/ml
18.2 ml	250 000 Units/ml

How much do you give the patient?

Note: Since the doctor has ordered 750 000 Units, choose to add 8.2 ml diluent to make a solution strength of 500 000 Units in 1 ml. This is the strength you will use in the dosage calculation. Notice that the amount to administer will be between 1 and 2 ml.

1. **Dosage Formula**

$$750\,000 \text{ U} \div \frac{500\,000 \text{ U}}{1 \text{ ml}} = 750\,000 \text{ U} \times \frac{1 \text{ ml}}{500\,000 \text{ U}} = \frac{750\,000}{500\,000} = 1.5 \text{ ml}$$

2. **DQA Proportion**

$$\frac{750\,000 \text{ U}}{500\,000 \text{ U}} = \frac{\text{X ml}}{1 \text{ ml}}$$

$$500\,000 \text{ X} = 750\,000$$

$$\text{X} = \frac{750\,000}{500\,000} = 1.5 \text{ ml}$$

3. **DHQ Formula**

$$\frac{750\,000 \text{ U}}{500\,000 \text{ U}} \times 1 \text{ ml} = 1.5 \text{ ml}$$

4. **Label Proportion**

$$\frac{750\,000\ \text{U}}{\text{X ml}} = \frac{500\,000\ \text{U}}{1\ \text{ml}}$$

$$500\,000\ \text{X} = 750\,000$$

$$\text{X} = \frac{750\,000}{500\,000} = 1.5\ \text{ml}$$

Answer: Give 1.5 ml penicillin G
                  Relabel the vial: 750 000 Units = 1.5 ml (500 000 U/ml)
                                              Date and time of preparation, and your initials.

Problems to try. Answers to these problems appear at the end of 7.3 exercises.

c. Ordered: 100 000 U q.a.m.

Label info:	Volume of Diluent	Concentration of Solution
	7.8 ml	50 000 U/ml
	5.6 ml	100 000 U/ml
	3.4 ml	200 000 U/ml

How much of what strength do you give the patient and how often?

d. Ordered: 75 000 U q.a.m.

Label info:	Volume of Diluent	Concentration of Solution
	7.8 ml	50 000 U/ml
	5.6 ml	100 000 U/ml
	3.4 ml	200 000 U/ml

How much of what strength do you give the patient and how often?

7.3   Exercises
---

a. Calculate the patient dosage;   b. Tell how often to give the dosage and;
c. State how to relabel the vial or if you should discard it. Remember, use
medication strength in dosage calculations.

1. Ordered: phenobarbital sodium   120 mg   IM   q.12h.
   Available: 2 ml vial containing 150 mg phenobarbital sodium powder

   a. _____

   b. _____

   c. _____

2. Ordered: ANCEF® (sterile cefazolin sodium [lyophilized])
                     500 mg IM q.12h.
   Available: 1 g vial; add 2.5 ml diluent. Approx. available vol. = 3 ml

   a. _____

   b. _____

   c. _____

3. Ordered: CHLOROMYCETIN®   100 mg   IM   q.6h.
   Available: 10 ml vial of powder labeled 1000 mg

   a. _____

   b. _____

   c. _____

4. Ordered: KEFZOL® (cefazolin sodium)   500 mg   IM   q.8h.
   Available: vial of powdered medication labeled "1 g KEFZOL®—add
                 2.5 ml sterile water to dissolve and produce a solution in which
                 1 ml = 300 mg."

   a. _____

   b. _____

   c. _____

5. Ordered: potassium penicillin G   1 500 000 U   IM   q.12h.
    Label: potassium penicillin G for injection, 5 000 000 U.

Preparation of Solution

Add Diluent	Concentration
18.2 ml	250 000 U/ml
8.2 ml	500 000 U/ml
3.2 ml	1 000 000 U/ml

    a. _____

    b. _____

    c. _____

6. Ordered: potassium penicillin G 100 000 U   IM   q.8h.
    Available: vial of powdered potassium penicillin G labled "1 000 000 U—
                   add 9.6 ml diluent to provide 100 000 U/ml;
                   add 4.6 ml diluent to provide 200 000 U/ml;
                   add 3.6 ml diluent to provide 250 000 U/ml"

    a. _____

    b. _____

    c. _____

7. Ordered: aqueous penicillin 500 000 U q.4h.
    Available: vial labeled "1 000 000 U—add 3.6 ml diluent to make each ml
                   equivalent to 250 000 U. Total volume 4 ml"

    a. _____

    b. _____

    c. _____

8. Ordered: MONOCID® 500 mg   IM   q.a.m.
    Label:

    > bulk vial   10 grams
    > **MONOCID®**
    > (sterile cefonicid sodium [lyophilized])
    > Dilute with 45 ml SW for injection
    > 1 g/5 ml   volume   51 ml

    a. _____

    b. _____

    c. _____

9. Ordered: MONOCID®   500   mg   IM   b.i.d.
    Label:

    > 500 mg vial
    > **MONOCID®**
    > (sterile cefonicid sodium [lyophilized])
    > Use 2.0 ml diluent
    > total volume 2.2 ml
    > 225 mg/ml

    a. _____

    b. _____

    c. _____

10. Ordered: MONOCID®   500 mg   IM   daily
    Label:

    > bulk vial   10 grams
    > **MONOCID®**
    > (sterile cefonicid sodium [lyophilized])
    > Dilute with 25 ml SW for injection
    > 1 g/3 ml   volume 31 ml

    a. _____

    b. _____

    c. _____

11.   Ordered: SOLU-MEDROL®   200 mg   IM   daily for 1 week
       Label:

---

2 gram vial
SOLU-MEDROL® Sterile Powder

methylprednisolone sodium succinate

30.6 ml volume when mixed with diluent

use within 48 hours after mixing

---

a. _____

b. _____

c. _____

12.   Ordered: SOLU-MEDROL®   80 mg   IM   q.o.d.
       Label:

---

500 mg vial
SOLU-MEDROL® Sterile Powder

methylprednisolone sodium succinate

8.0 ml volume when mixed with diluent

use within 48 hours after mixing

---

a. _____

b. _____

c. _____

13.   Ordered: PIPRACIL®   500 mg   IM   t.i.d.
       Label:

PIPRACIL®   2 gram vial

piperacillin sodium

add 2 ml sterile water for injection

1 g = 2.5 ml

---

a. _____

b. _____

c. _____

14. Ordered: TAZICEF®   250 mg   IM   q.12h.
     Label:

> 6 gram bulk vial
> **TAZICEF®**
> (ceftazidime) for injection
> 26 ml diluent   volume 30 ml

  a. _____

  b. _____

  c. _____

15. Ordered: TAZICEF®   30 mg/kg body mass   IV   q.8h.
     Child's weight: 22 pounds
     Label:

> 6 gram bulk vial
> **TAZICEF®**
> (ceftazidime) for injection
> 26 ml diluent   volume 30 ml

  a. _____

  b. _____

  c. _____

16. Ordered: ANCEF®   500 mg   IM   t.i.d.
     Label:

> **ANCEF®**   1 gram
> (sterile cefazolin sodium [lyophilized])
> Diluent 2.5 ml   Volume 3 ml
> 330 mg/ml

  a. _____

  b. _____

  c. _____

17. Ordered: ANCEF®   500 mg   IM   q.8h.
     Label:

> ANCEF®   5 gram bulk vial
>
> (sterile cefazolin sodium [lyophilized])
>
> Diluent 23 ml   Volume 26 ml
>
> 1 g/5 ml

a. _____

b. _____

c. _____

18. Ordered: CEFIZOX®   500 mg   q.12h.
     Label:

> 1 gram vial
>
> CEFIZOX®
>
> (sterile ceftizoxime sodium)
>
> 3 ml diluent   3.7 ml volume
>
> 270 mg/ml

a. _____

b. _____

c. _____

19. Ordered: CEFIZOX®   50 mg/kg   body mass   q.6h.
     Patient weight: 17 pounds
     Label:

> 1 gram vial
>
> CEFIZOX®
>
> (sterile ceftizoxime sodium)
>
> 3 mil diluent   3.7 ml volume
>
> 270 mg/ml

a. _____

b. _____

c. _____

20. Ordered: ANCEF®   250 mg   IM   q.i.d.
     Label:

> **ANCEF®   5 gram bulk vial**
> (sterile cefazolin sodium [lyophilized])
> Diluent 23 ml   Volume 26 ml
> **1 g/5 ml**

a. _____

b. _____

c. _____

Answers to Problems to try.

a. 1.5 ml IM every day at 10 a.m.; discard vial
b. 0.5 ml IM three times a day; date, time, and initials on label
c. 1 ml of 100 000 U/ml strength in the morning; date, time, and initials on label
d. 1.5 ml of 50 000 U/ml strength in the morning; date, time, and initials on label

---

Space Provided for Student Work

7.4   Calculating the Amount of Medication in a Solution

To determine the amount of pure medication, by weight, in a solution with a specified strength, use one of the dosage calculation formulas with the medication weight as the unknown. The strength of a pure medication is 100%. Recall that strengths stated as a % or ratio always refer to grams per milliliter.

Example: How much sodium bicarbonate is contained in 500 ml of a 5% IV solution?

Note: Recall that 5% strength means 5 grams in 100 ml

1. **Dosage Formula**

$$500 \text{ ml} \div \frac{100 \text{ ml}}{5 \text{ g}} = 500 \text{ ml} \times \frac{5 \text{ g}}{100 \text{ ml}} = \frac{2500}{100} \text{ g} = 25 \text{ g}$$

2. **DQA Proportion**

$$\frac{5 \text{ g}}{X \text{ g}} = \frac{100 \text{ ml}}{500 \text{ ml}}$$

$$100 \, X = 2500$$

$$X = 25 \text{ g}$$

3. **DHQ Formula**

$$\frac{500 \text{ ml}}{100 \text{ ml}} \times 5 \text{ g} = \frac{2500}{100} \text{ g} = 25 \text{ g}$$

4. **Label Proportion**

$$\frac{X \text{ g}}{500 \text{ ml}} = \frac{5 \text{ g}}{100 \text{ ml}}$$

$$100 \, X = 2500$$

$$X = 25 \text{ g}$$

Answer: There are 25 g of sodium bicarbonate in 500 ml of a 5% solution.

7.4   Exercises

Determine the amount of pure medication, by weight, in the following solutions.

1. How many grams of potassium citrate (crystals) are contained in 50 ml of 7% potassium citrate solution?

2. How many grams of epinephrine (solids) are contained in 1.5 liters of 1:1000 epinephrine solution?

3. How many grams of crystalline glucose are contained in 200 ml of 1:10 glucose solution?

4. How many grams of sodium chloride are contained in 500 ml of 0.9% saline solution?

5. How many mg of powdered bichloride of mercury are contained in 100 ml of 1:500 bichloride of mercury solution?

6. How many mg of a medication would be needed to prepare 1500 ml of 1:5000 solution?

7. How many ml of solution strength 1 g/20 ml can be made from 0.3 g of silver nitrate?

8. How many grams of sodium chloride are contained in 1 liter of half-strength (0.45%) saline solution?

9. How many liters of saline solution (0.9%) can be made from 18 g of sodium chloride?

10. How many grams of boric acid crystals are needed to prepare 150 ml of 5% boric acid solution?

11. How many ml of 2% cocaine solution can be made from 500 mg of crystalline cocaine?

Space Provided for Student Work

7.5   Diluting Solutions

Sometimes it is necessary to dilute a concentrated solution to a weaker concentration (strength). The strength of the solution may be listed as a percent or a ratio (the formulas below show % but ratios may be substituted). Dilution of solutions requires an arithmetic process called "inverse variation" or "inverse proportion." There are two acceptable methods of solving problems using inverse variation.

1. **Inverse Proportion**
    This proportion is set up with the given strength and volume in the means, and the desired strength and volume in the extremes. Therefore, the labeled strength is not together on one side of the proportion.

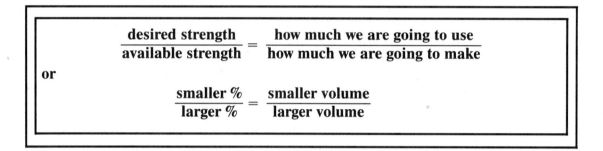

$$\frac{\text{desired strength}}{\text{available strength}} = \frac{\text{how much we are going to use}}{\text{how much we are going to make}}$$

or

$$\frac{\text{smaller \%}}{\text{larger \%}} = \frac{\text{smaller volume}}{\text{larger volume}}$$

2. **Dilution Equation**
    This equation is the result of multiplying cross products in the inverse proportion above; however, it is easier to set up and use because the label strength and volume are both contained on the same side of the equation. The other side contains the desired strength and dosage.

    (available volume)(label strength) = (dosage volume)(desired strength)
    or

    strong solution = weak solution
    (given vol.)(%) = (final volume)(%)

The answer to a dilution problem should state the number of ml of concentrate needed, and the final volume and diluted strength.

Example: A medication of 50% strength is to be diluted with sterile water to make a 20% strength solution. How much sterile water should be added to the concentrated solution to prepare 100 ml of 20% solution?

1. **Inverse Proportion**

    $$\frac{20\%}{50\%} = \frac{X \text{ ml}}{100 \text{ ml}}$$

    $$50 X = 2000$$

    $$X = \frac{2000}{50} = 40 \text{ ml}$$

2. **Dilution Equation**

    $$(100 \text{ ml})(20\%) = (X \text{ ml})(50\%)$$

    $$2000 = 50 X$$

    $$X = \frac{2000}{50} = 40 \text{ ml}$$

Answer: To prepare 100 ml of 20% solution, take 40 ml of 50% solution and add 60 ml sterile water to make a total of 100 ml.

Example: How many ml of 1:100 potassium permanganate solution are needed to prepare 1000 ml of 1:8000 potassium permanganate sclution?

1. **Inverse Proportion**

    $$\frac{1:8000}{1:100} = \frac{X \text{ ml}}{1000 \text{ ml}}$$

    $$\frac{1}{8000}(1000) = \frac{1}{100}(X) \qquad \text{Cross multiply.}$$

    $$\frac{1}{8} = \frac{X}{100} \qquad \text{Simplify.}$$

    $$8 X = 100 \qquad \text{Cross multiply.}$$

    $$X = \frac{100}{8} = 12.5 \text{ ml}$$

2. **Dilution Equation**

    $$(X \text{ ml})(1:100) = (1000 \text{ ml})(1:8000)$$

    $$\frac{X}{1}\left(\frac{1}{100}\right) = \frac{1000}{1}\left(\frac{1}{8000}\right)$$

    $$\frac{X}{100} = \frac{1}{8} \qquad \text{Simplify.}$$

    $$8 X = 100 \qquad \text{Cross multiply.}$$

    $$X = 12.5 \text{ ml}$$

Answer: To prepare 1000 ml of 1:8000 solution, take 12.5 ml of 1:100 solution and add 987.5 ml diluent to make a total of 1000 ml.

Example: Prepare 500 ml of 1:50 (or 2% strength) formaldehyde solution from a 40% solution of formaldehyde.

1. **Inverse Proportion**

$$\frac{2\%}{40\%} = \frac{X\,ml}{500\,ml}$$

$$40\,X = 2(500)$$

$$X = \frac{1000}{40} = 25\,ml$$

2. **Dilution Equation**

$$(40\%)(X\,ml) = (2\%)(500\,ml)$$

$$40X = 1000$$

$$X = \frac{1000}{40} = 25\,ml$$

Answer: To prepare 500 ml of 1:50 formaldehyde solution, take 25 ml of 40% solution and add 475 ml sterile water to make a total of 500 ml.

Problems to try. Answers to these problems appear at the end of 7.5 exercises.

a. How many ml of a 20% solution are needed to prepare 50 ml of a 5% solution?

b. How many ml of a 1:10000 solution are needed to prepare 500 ml of a 1:20000 solution?

7.5   *Exercises*

When answering the following problems, state the volume of the given concentrate to be used, the volume of diluent to be added, and the final volume and diluted strength of the desired solution.

1. ZEPHIRAN® Chloride (benzalkonium chloride) antiseptic is available in a 17% concentration. How many ml of this concentration are needed to prepare 500 ml of 0.1% solution?

2. How many liters of a 1:10000 solution do you need to prepare 2 liters of a 1:20000 solution?

3. Concentrated sodium chloride solution has a strength of 23.4%. How many ml would you add to sterile water to prepare 100 ml of normal saline solution (0.9% strength)?

4. How many ml of concentrated sodium chloride solution (23.4% strength) would you add to sterile water to prepare 500 ml of half-strength saline solution (0.45% strength)?

5. How many ml of 2:5 solution are needed to prepare 2000 ml of 4% solution?

6. The surgical nursing station calls and asks for 10 liters of benzalkonium chloride 1:1000 for instrument cleaning. How many ml of benzalkonium chloride 17% would you need to prepare each liter of the solution?

7. The inhalation therapist has a requisition for 120 ml of 70% ethyl alcohol. You have a bottle of 95% ethyl alcohol. Calculate the amount of 95% ethyl alcohol needed to prepare 120 ml of 70% ethyl alcohol.

8. How many ml of pure liquid cresol (100%) are needed to prepare 300 ml of 2% cresol solution?

9. How many ml of 10% solution are needed to prepare 20 ml of 1:100 solution?

10. How many ml of pure glucose (100%) are needed to make 1 liter of 5% glucose solution?

11.   Calculate the amount in ounces of 6% vinegar (acetic acid) needed to prepare a gallon of 0.25% acetic acid solution.

12.   Change 0.02% to a ratio strength.

13.   Change $\frac{8\,g}{50\,ml}$ to a percent strength.

14.   Change 1:500 to a percent strength.

15.   Change 1:2000 to a percent strength.

16.   Change 0.9% to a ratio strength.

17.   How many ml of 2% mercurochrome solution are needed to prepare 250 ml of 1% mercurochrome solution?

18.   How many ml of nitrofurazone 0.1% solution can be prepared from 450 ml of Nitrofurazone 0.2% solution?

19.   Prepare 200 ml cupric sulfate 1:4000 for use as a fungicidal agent. Cupric sulfate 5% is available. How many ml of concentrate are needed?

Answers to Problems to try.

a. To prepare 50 ml of 5% solution, take 12.5 ml of 20% solution and add 37.5 ml diluent.

b. To prepare 500 ml of a 1:20000 solution, take 250 ml of a 1:10000 solution and add 250 ml diluent.

7.6   Calculating Pediatric Dosages by Body Weight

Children's dosages are calculated according to the amount of medication per body weight. Labels are usually written as mg/kg/day, but you might also see mg/lb./day.

A label that reads **50 mg/kg/day** would mean that you would administer 50 mg medication for every kg of body weight in a period of one day.

TO CALCULATE CHILDREN'S DOSAGE USING BODY WEIGHT:
1a. if the medication is per kg of body weight, then the child's weight must be in kilograms; round to tenths;
1b. if the medication is per lb. of body weight, then the child's weight must be in pounds; round to tenths;
2. multiply the label by the child's weight.

$$\frac{mg}{kg} \times kg \qquad or \qquad \frac{mg}{lb.} \times lb.$$

Example: Ordered: amoxicillin for a child weighing 15 kg
Label: amoxicillin 20 mg/kg/day in divided dosages q.8h.
How many mg can the child receive in one day?
How many mg can the child receive in one dose?

The child's weight is already in kilograms; substitute the information into the formula and solve.

$$\frac{20\ mg}{1\ kg} \times 15\ kg = \text{multiply the label by the body weight}$$

$$20 \times 15 = 300\ mg/day \qquad 300 \div 3 = 100\ mg/dose$$

Example: Ordered: KEFLEX® for a child weighing 29 lb.
Label: KEFLEX® (cephalexin) 25 mg/lb./day
How many mg can the child receive in one day?

The child's weight is already in pounds; substitute the information into the formula and solve.

$$\frac{25 \text{ mg}}{1 \text{ lb.}} \times 29 \text{ lb} = 25 \times 29 = 725 \text{ mg/day}$$

Example: Ordered: medication for a child weighing 12 kg
Label: 100 mg/kg/day can be given q.6h.
How many mg can the child receive in one day?
How many mg can the child receive in each dose?

The child's weight is already in kilograms; substitute the information into the formula and solve.

$$\frac{100 \text{ mg}}{1 \text{ kg}} \times 12 \text{ kg} = 100 \times 20 = 1200 \text{ mg/day}$$

The child can receive 4 doses per day (q.6h.).

Divide the dosage per day by the number of doses.

$$1200 \div 4 = 300 \text{ mg/dose}$$

Example: Ordered: ILOSONE® (erythromycin estolate) 30 mg/kg/day to be given q.6h.
The child weighs 15 lb.
How many mg can the child receive in one day?
How many mg can the child receive each dose?

Since the child's weight is in pounds and the label is per kg, you need to first convert pounds to kilograms (1 kg = 2.2 lb.).

$$15 \text{ lb.} \times \frac{1 \text{ kg}}{2.2 \text{ lb.}} = \frac{15}{2.2} = 6.8 \text{ kg}$$

Substitute the information into the formula and solve.

$$\frac{30 \text{ mg}}{1 \text{ kg}} \times 6.8 \text{ kg} = 30 \times 6.8 = 204 \text{ mg/day}$$

The child can receive 4 doses/day, so divide the dosage per day by 4.

$$204 \div 4 = 51 \text{ mg per dose}$$

The answer may not always come out to an even number. The physician will order the amount of medication to be given, but you will need to determine if the dose ordered is within a safe range for the child.

Problems to try. Answers to these problems appear at the end of 7.6 exercises.

a. Ordered: antibiotic q.4h. for a 5 kg infant
   Label: antibiotic 60 mg/kg/day

   How many mg can the child receive in one day?   _____

   How many mg can the child receive per dose?   _____

b. Ordered: medication t.i.d. for 66 lb child
   Label: medication 30 mg/kg/day

   How many mg can the child receive in one day?   _____

   How many mg can the child receive in each dose?   _____

7.6   *Exercises*

---

1.   Ordered: ANCEF® q.i.d. to 20 lb. child
     Label: ANCEF® (sterile cefazolin sodium [lyophilized] 100 mg/kg/day)

     How many mg can the child receive in one day?   _____

     How many mg can the child receive in every dose?   _____

2.   Ordered: KEFLEX® q.8h. to 24 lb. child
     Label: KEFLEX® (cephalexin) 25 mg/kg/day

     How many mg can the child receive in one day?   _____

     How many mg can the child receive in each dose?   _____

3.   Ordered: DEMEROL® 0.5 mg/lb. to be given one time to a 30 lb. child
     Label: DEMEROL® (meperidine hydrochloride) 50 mg/ml

     How many ml will you administer?   _____

4.   Ordered: CHLOROMYCETIN® 25 mg/kg/day, given in divided
          doses q.8h.
     Child's weight: 17 lbs.

     How many mg can the child receive in one day?   _____

     How many mg can the child receive in every dose?   _____

5.   Ordered: ampicillin 50 mg/kg/day to be given in divided doses q.6h.
     Child's weight: 19 lbs.

     How many mg can the child receive in one dose?   _____

6.   Ordered: OMNIPEN® q.i.d. to 26.4 lb. child
     Label: OMNIPEN® (ampicillin) Oral Suspension 50 mg/kg/day

     How many mg can the child receive in one day?   _____

     How many mg can the child receive per dose?   _____

7.   Ordered: KLONOPIN® (clonazepam) 0.01 mg/kg/day to be given q.8h.
     Child's weight: 21 lbs.

     How many mg can the child receive in one day?   _____

     How many mg can the child receive in each dose?   _____

8.   Ordered: OMNIPEN® (ampicillin) 50 mg/kg/day to be given q.6h.
     Child's weight: 17 lbs.

     How many mg can the child receive in one day?   _____

     How many mg can the child receive in every dose?   _____

9. Ordered: ELIXOPHYLLIN® (theophylline anhydrous) 6 mg/kg as an initial dose.
    Child's weight: 52 lbs.

    How many mg can the child receive in one dose?   _____

10. Ordered: ELIXOPHYLLIN® (theophylline anhydrous) 4 mg/kg to be given q.4h. for three doses.
     Child's weight: 52 lbs.

     How many mg can the child receive in each dose?   _____

11. Ordered: CECLOR® (cefaclor) 20 mg/kg/day to be given in divided doses q.8h.
     Child's weight: 18 lbs.

     How many mg can the child receive in one day?   _____

     How many mg can the child receive per dose?   _____

12. Ordered: VANCOCIN® (vancomycin hydrochloride) 40 mg/kg/day to be given q.6h.
     Child's weight: 82 lbs.

     How many mg can the child receive in one day?   _____

     How many mg can the child receive in every dose?   _____

13. Ordered: Children's PANADOL® (acetaminophen) 10 mg/kg each dose. May be given q.i.d.
     Child's weight: 50 lbs.

     How many mg can the child receive in one dose?   _____

14.   Ordered: GANTRISIN® (sulfisoxazole) 150 mg/kg/day to be given in 4 divided doses.
Child's weight: 21 lbs.

How many mg can the child receive in one day?   _____

How many mg can the child receive in each dose?   _____

15.   Ordered: KEFLEX® (cephalexin) 25 mg/kg/day to be given in divided doses q.8h.
Child's weight: 34 lbs.

How many mg can the child receive in one day?   _____

How many mg can the child receive in every dose?   _____

Answers to Problems to try.

a. 300 mg, 50 mg   b. 900 mg, 300 mg

Space Provided for Student Work

7.7   *Dosage Calculation Using a Nomogram*

Another way to calculate patient dosage is by finding the patient's **body surface area** (**BSA**) using a nomogram. To use a nomogram you must know the patient's height and weight.

Dosage calculations using BSA are considered by some to be more accurate than body weight calculations. Although you may not be required to calculate the dosage, you will be responsible for checking to see if the dosage is within safe limits.

First, look at the nomogram on page 209. Notice that there are different intervals between the labeled marks on the same scale.

TO FIND THE VALUES OF THE UNLABELED MARKS ON A SCALE:
   a. **calculate the distance between two labeled marks;**
   b. **count the spaces between these two marks;**
   c. **divide the distance by the number of spaces.**

Look at the "Height" column first. The height column is in feet and centimeters.

Height column—feet

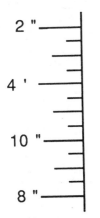

The distance between each labeled mark is 2″.
Between each labeled mark there are 4 spaces.
So each unlabeled mark represents $\frac{2″}{4}$ or $\frac{1}{2}$ inch.

Convert inches to feet and inches by dividing by 12 (12 inches = 1 ft.).

Example: $52″ = 4′4″$

Examples: a. Find $45\frac{1}{2}''$

              b. Find 3'11''

              c. Find $4'\frac{1}{2}''$

              d. Find 50''

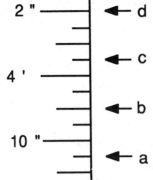

Height column—centimeters

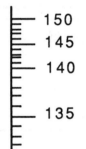

The distance between each labeled mark is 5 cm. Even though the physical distance gets smaller as you go up the scale, there are always 5 spaces between each labeled mark. So each unlabeled mark represents $\frac{5\ cm}{5}$ or 1 cm.

Examples: a. Find 137 cm

                b. Find 134 cm

                c. Find 148 cm

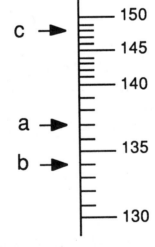

The "Surface Area" column is in square meters (m²).

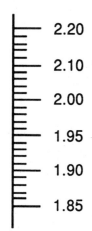

The distance between each labeled mark on this scale changes. Below 2.00 m² the distance is 0.05 m² with 5 spaces between. So each mark represents $\frac{0.05 \text{ m}^2}{5}$ or 0.01 m².

Above 2.00 m² the distance is 0.1 m² with 5 spaces between. So each mark represents $\frac{0.1 \text{ m}^2}{5}$ or 0.02 m².

Examples: a. Find 1.97 m²
b. Find 1.92 m²
c. Find 2.08 m²
d. Find 2.16 m²
e. Find 1.86 m²

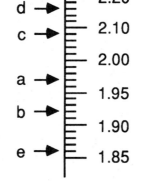

The "Weight" column is in pounds and kilograms.

Weight column—pounds

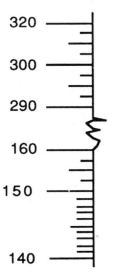

Both the distance between and the number of spaces between each labeled mark change.

Below 150 lbs. the distance is 10 lbs. and the number of spaces between is 10. So each mark represents $\frac{10 \text{ lbs.}}{10}$ or 1 lb.

From 150 to 300 lbs. the distance is 10 lbs. and the number of spaces is 4. So each mark represents $\frac{10 \text{ lbs.}}{4}$ or $2\frac{1}{2}$ lb.

Above 300 lb. the distance is 20 lb. and the number of spaces is 4. So each mark represents $\frac{20 \text{ lbs.}}{4}$ or 5 lbs.

KVCG KALAMAZOO VALLEY COMMUNITY COLLEGE LIBRARY

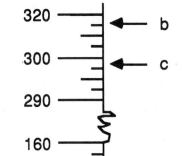

Examples: a. Find 146 lbs.
b. Find 315 lbs.
c. Find 298 lbs.
d. Find 152 lbs.

Weight column-kilogram

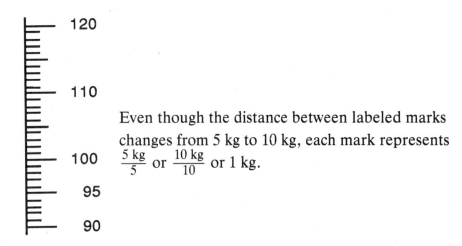

Even though the distance between labeled marks changes from 5 kg to 10 kg, each mark represents $\frac{5 \text{ kg}}{5}$ or $\frac{10 \text{ kg}}{10}$ or 1 kg.

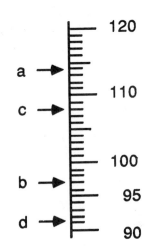

Examples: a. Find 114 kg
b. Find 97 kg
c. Find 108 kg
d. Find 91 kg

NOMOGRAM
(Courtesy Abbott Laboratories)

HEIGHT		SURFACE AREA	WEIGHT	
feet	centimeters	in square meters	pounds	kilograms

HEIGHT (feet)	HEIGHT (centimeters)	SURFACE AREA (in square meters)	WEIGHT (pounds)	WEIGHT (kilograms)
			440	200
			420	190
			400	180
			380	170
			360	160
			340	150
			320	140
7′	220	3.00	300	
10″	215	2.90	290	130
8″	210	2.80	280	
6″	205	2.70	270	120
4″	200	2.60	260	
2″	195	2.50	250	
	190	2.40	240	110
6′	185	2.30	230	
10″	180	2.20	220	100
8″	175	2.10	210	95
6″	170	2.00	200	90
4″	165	1.95	190	85
2″	160	1.90	180	80
5′	155	1.85	170	75
	150	1.80	160	
10″	145	1.75	150	70
8″	140	1.70	140	65
6″	135	1.65	130	60
4″	130	1.60	120	55
2″	125	1.55	110	50
4′	120	1.50	100	45
10″	115	1.45	90	40
8″	110	1.40	80	35
6″	105	1.35	70	30
4′	100	1.30	60	25
2″	95	1.25	50	20
3′	90	1.20		
10″	85	1.15		
8″	80	1.10		
6″	75	1.05		

Now that you can read each scale, use the nomogram to find the BSA given the patient's height and weight.

Example: Patient's height is 148 cm and weight is 37 kg.
What is the patient's BSA in m²?

Find 148 cm on the height scale.
Find 37 kg on the weight scale.
Using a rule draw a line between these two points.
This line cross the surface area scale at 1.25 m².

Example: Patient's height is 57″ and weight is 99 lbs.
What is the patient's BSA in m²?

Find 57″ on the height scale.
Find 99 lbs. on the weight scale.
Using a ruler draw a line between these two points.
This line crosses the surface area scale at 1.33 m².

If the line crosses the surface area scale between two marks, choose the smaller BSA.

Problems to try. Answers to these problems appear at the end of 7.7 exercises.

a. Patient height: 45″
   Patient weight: 26 kg
   Patient BSA: _____

b. Patient height: 6′4″
   Patient weight: 255 lbs.
   Patient BSA: _____

In calculating patient dosage using BSA, the label will read "mg per m²" (mg/m²). Solve these problems by using either a Proportion or the Factor-label method.

Example: Patient height: 5′
Patient weight: 105 lbs.
Label: 65 mg/m²
Calculate patient's BSA and dosage.

From the nomogram, BSA is 1.42 m^2.

1. **Proportion**

$$\frac{65 \text{ mg}}{1 \text{ m}^2} = \frac{X \text{ mg}}{1.42 \text{ m}^2}$$

$$X = 65(1.42) = 92.3 \quad \text{or} \quad 92 \text{ mg}$$

2. **Factor-label**

$$\frac{65 \text{ mg}}{1 \text{ m}^2} \times 1.42 \text{ m}^2 = 65(1.42) = 92.3 \quad \text{or} \quad 92 \text{ mg}$$

Example: Patient height: 100 cm
Patient weight: 24 kg
Label: 30 mg/m^2
Calculate patient's BSA and dosage.

From the nomogram, BSA is 0.79 m^2.

1. **Proportion**

$$\frac{30 \text{ mg}}{1 \text{ m}^2} = \frac{X \text{ mg}}{0.79 \text{ m}^2}$$

$$X = 30(0.79) = 23.7 \quad \text{or} \quad 24 \text{ mg}$$

2. **Factor-label**

$$\frac{30 \text{ mg}}{1 \text{ m}^2} \times 0.79 \text{ m}^2 = 30(0.79) = 23.7 \quad \text{or} \quad 24 \text{ mg}$$

Problems to try. Answers to these problems appear at the end of 7.7 exercises.

c. Patient height: 56″
   Patient weight: 46 kg
   Label: 70 mg/m^2

   Patient BSA: _____

   Patient dosage: _____

d. Patient height: 95 cm
   Patient weight: 49 lbs.
   Label: 30 mg/m^2

Patient BSA: _____

Patient dosage: _____

7.7 Exercises

Use the nomogram on page 209 to find the patient's BSA in m^2.

1. Patient height: 162 cm
   Patient weight: 140 lbs.

   Patient BSA: _____

2. Patient height: 60″
   Patient weight: 89 kg

   Patient BSA: _____

3. Patient height: 6′8″
   Patient weight: 182 lbs.

   Patient BSA: _____

4. Patient height: 83 cm
   Patient weight: 21 kg

   Patient BSA _____

5. Patient height: 4′3$\frac{1}{2}$″
   Patient weight: 66 lbs.

   Patient BSA: _____

In the following problems: a. find the patient's BSA using the nomogram; and b. calculate the patient dosage.

6. Ordered: ONCOVIN® (vincristine sulfate) 2 mg/m² IV weekly
   The child is 48 inches tall and weighs 50 lbs.

   a. _____

   b. _____

7. Ordered: ONCOVIN® (vincristine sulfate) 2 mg/m² IV weekly
   The child is 58 inches tall and weighs 75 lbs.

   a. _____

   b. _____

8. Ordered: ADRIAMYCIN PFS® (doxorubicin hydrochloride) 60 mg/m² as
   a one-time dose
   The patient is 60 inches tall and weighs 55 kg.

   a. _____

   b. _____

9. Ordered: ADRIAMYCIN PFS® (doxorubicin hydrochloride) 20 mg/m²
   weekly
   The patient is 57″ tall and weighs 105 lbs.

   a. _____

   b. _____

10. Ordered: ZOVIRAX® (acyclovir) 250 mg/m² q.8h.
    The patient is 163 cm tall and weighs 64 kg.

    a. _____

    b. _____

11. Ordered: ZOVIRAX® (acyclovir) 250 mg/m² q.8h.
    The patient is 6 ft. tall and weighs 180 lbs.

    a. _____

    b. _____

12. Ordered: ADRIAMYCIN PFS® (doxorubicin hydrochloride) 30 mg/m²
    The patient is 40″ tall and weighs 52 lbs.

    a. _____

    b. _____

13. Ordered: ADRIAMYCIN PFS® (doxorubicin hydrochloride) 60 mg/m²
             q.21 days
    The patient is 63″ tall and weighs 115 lbs.

    a. _____

    b. _____

Answers to Problems to try.

a. 0.88 m²   b. 2.44 m²   c. 132 m², 92.4 mg   d. 0.72 m², 21.6 mg

Chapter 7 Test

Interpret medication strength from this label information:

1. 40%   _____

2. 1:100   _____

3. U-100   _____

4. 25 mg = 2 cc   _____

5. 40 mEq/30 ml   _____

6.

20 dosette vials—each contains 1 ml
MORPHINE SULFATE
INJECTION, USP
15 mg/ml

7.

20 ml vial
ATROPINE SULFATE
INJECTION, USP
0.4 mg (1/50 gr.) per ml

Calculate the patient dosage needed to fill the doctor's orders.

8. Ordered: insulin 30 U
   Available: U-100 insulin and a syringe marked in cc
   How many cc's do you administer?_____

9. Ordered: 220 mg q.i.d.
   Available: vial labeled 30% strength solution
   How many ml do you give?_____

10. Ordered: 550 mg IM b.i.d.
    Label: "8.2 g—inject 20.5 ml sterile water to yield 30 ml"
    How many ml do you give?_____

11. Ordered: 80 mg
    Available: 2 cc ampule labeled 330 mg
    How many cc's do you give?   _____

12. How many ml of U-100 insulin are needed to give 45 units?   _____

13. Ordered: 150 mg P.O. q.p.m.
    Available: 1:30 solution
    How many ml do you give?   _____

14. Ordered: KCL 15 mEq to IV fluids
    Label: 20 mEq/10 ml
    How many ml will you add to the IV fluids?   _____

15. Ordered: gr. viiss
    Label: 30% solution
    How many ml do you use?   _____

16. Ordered: 80 000 U ampicillin q.6h.
    Label info: the vial insert reads:

Volume of Diluent	Concentration
6.8 ml	60 000 U/ml
4.2 ml	120 000 U/ml
2.0 ml	200 000 U/ml

    How many ml of which strength do you give?   _____

17. How many ounces of 70% sorbital solution would you use if the doctor ordered 4 oz. of 30% sorbital solution? How many ml would you use?

18. Ordered: gr. xvi t.i.d.
    Label: 7% solution
    How many ml do you give per dose?_____

19. How many ml of pure glucose (100%) are needed to make 5 liters of 9% glucose solution?

20. Ordered: chlorprothixene liquid 40 mg t.i.d.
    Label:

    > 1 gram vial
    > TARACTAN® LIQUID
    > (Chlorprothixene lactate and HCL)
    > 5 ml = 100 mg

    Patient dosage: _____

21. Ordered: thioridazine liquid 0.1 g
    Label:

    > 20 ml vial
    > MELLARIL® LIQUID
    > (thioridazine)
    > 1 ml = 30 mg

    Patient dosage:_____

22. Ordered: Garamycin® 65 mg   IM
    Label:

    > multidose vial
    > GARAMYCIN® Injectable
    > (gentamicin sulfate)
    > 40 mg/ml

    Patient dosage: _____

23. Ordered: chloral hydrate liquid 0.75 g
    Label: solution of strength 1 f ℨ = 0.5 g
    How many oz. do you give? _____

24. Ordered: medication 300 μg IM
    Available: vial labeled 0.4 mg/0.5 ml
    How many ml do you give? _____

25. How many ccs are needed to give 50 units of U-100 insulin? _____

26. Ordered: penicillin G potassium   400 000 U   IM
    Label: buffered potassium penicillin G for injection, 5 000 000 U.

Preparation of Solution

Add Diluent	Concentration
18.2 ml	250 000 U/ml
8.2 ml	500 000 U/ml
3.2 ml	1 000 000 U/ml

How much of which strength do you give? _____

27. Ordered: magnesium sulfate 100 mg/kg of body mass
    Patient weight: 128 lbs.
    Label: 50% strength solution
    How many ml do you give? _____

28. Ordered: potassium iodide 400 mg
    Label: 30 ml dropper bottle labeled: 100 g:100 ml; each drop = $\frac{1}{10}$ ml
    How many drops do you administer? _____

29.   Ordered: morphine sulfate 10 mg   IM
      Label:

> 20 dosette vials—each contains 1 ml
> **MORPHINE SULFATE**
> INJECTION, USP
> 15 mg/ml

Patient dosage: _____

30.   Ordered: ANCEF® (sterile cefazolin sodium [lyophilized]) 1 g IM
      Available: 10 ml vial containing 5 grams
      How many ml do you give?   _____

31.   Ordered: Children's PANADOL® (acetaminophen) 10 mg/kg body
                     weight. May be given up to 5 times per day.
      Child's weight: 26 lbs.
      How many mg should the child receive per dose?   _____

32.   Ordered: DEMEROL® 0.5 mg/lb. to be given pre-operatively
      Child's weight: 40 lbs.
      Label: DEMEROL® (meperidine hydrochloride) 50 mg/ml
      How many mg should the child receive?   _____

      How many ml should the child receive?   _____

33.   Ordered: ILOSONE® (erythromycin estolate) 30 mg/kg/day to be
                     given q.6h.
      Child's weight: 17 lbs.
      How many mg should the child receive in one day?   _____

      How many mg should the child receive per dose?   _____

34. Ordered: CECLOR® (cefaclor) 20 mg/kg/day to be given in divided
        doses q.8h.
     Child's weight: 28 lbs.
     How many mg should the child receive in one day? _____

     How many mg should the child receive in each dose? _____

35. Ordered: KEFLEX® (cephalexin) 25 mg/kg/day to be given q.8h.
     Child's weight: 22 lbs.
     How many mg can the child receive in one day? _____

     How many mg can the child receive every dose? _____

36. Ordered: ADRIAMYCIN PFS® (doxorubicin hydrochloride) IM
     Patient's height and weight: 66 in.; 140 lbs.
     Label: 60 mg/m^2
     How many mg should be given per dose? _____

37. Ordered: ONCOVIN® (vincristine sulfate) IV weekly
     Patient's height and weight: 46 in.; 50 lbs.
     Label: 2 mg/m^2
     How many mg should be given per dose? _____

38. Ordered: ZOVIRAX® (acyclovir) q.8h.
     Patient's height and weight: 63 in.; 145 lbs.
     Label: 250 mg/m^2
     How many mg should be given per dose? _____

Chapter 8

IV Rates

This chapter explains how to calculate IV rates of flow. When you complete this chapter you should be able to:

a. Calculate rate of flow using the formula method or division factor method.
b. Find the total time an IV will run.
c. Calculate pediatric IVs.
d. Calculate piggyback rates of flow.
e. Calculate drug infusion rates.

8.1   Rate of Flow—Formula Method

IV (intravenous) fluids are usually ordered by the volume of fluid in milliliters to be given (infused) in a stated amount of time.

Examples: 1000 ml to be given in 8 hours
125 ml/hr.
3000 ml in 24 hours

The volume ordered is administered by adjusting the rate of flow (or flow rate) of the solution to be given. This is done by counting the drops per minute (gtts./min.).

The size of the drops is regulated by the **size of the IV tubing**. You will routinely see two types of IV tubing: the **standard** tubing is for use in most routine adult infusions; the **mini** or **micro** drip tubing is used when more exact measurement is needed. IV tubings are calibrated in drops per milliliter (gtts./ml).

With the standard IV tubing, 10, 15, or 20 drips is equal to 1 ml, depending on the type used. The mini or micro drip tubing will yield 60 drops to equal 1 ml. This information will be printed on the IV tubing package and is essential for calculating the flow rate.

The Formula Method

To calculate the flow rate you need the following information:

    a. the total volume of fluid to be infused in ml;
    b. the calibration of the tubing (also called drop factor);
    c. the time (in minutes) ordered for the infusion.

$$\frac{\textbf{Volume (ml)} \times \textbf{Calibration (gtts./ ml)}}{\textbf{Time (minutes)}} = \textbf{Flow Rate (gtts./ min.)}$$

Round your answers to the nearest whole number.

Example: Ordered: IV 5% D/W (dextrose in water) 150 ml/hr.
        Tubing calibration: 15 gtts./ml
        What is the flow rate?

$\dfrac{150 \text{ ml} \times 15 \text{ gtts./ml}}{1 \text{ hr. (60 min.)}}$ substitute information into the formula

$\dfrac{150 \times 15}{60} = \dfrac{2250}{60}$ do the multiplication first

$2250 \div 60 = 37.5$ then divide

38 gtts./min.   round and label your answer

Example: Ordered: IV 0.9% Saline 100 ml/30 min.
        Tubing drop factor: 10 gtts./ml
        What is the flow rate?

$$\frac{100 \text{ ml} \times 10 \text{ gtts./ml}}{30 \text{ min.}} = \frac{1000}{30} = 33.3 = 33 \text{ gtts./min.}$$

Example: Ordered: IV N.S. (normal Saline) 20 ml/30 min.
        Tubing drop factor: 60 gtts./ml
        What is the rate of flow?

$$\frac{20 \text{ ml} \times 60 \text{ gtts./ml}}{30 \text{ min.}} = \frac{1200}{30} = 40 \text{ gtts./min.}$$

Factor-Label Method

The Factor-Label Method used in conversions is mathematically equivalent to the Formula Method and may also be used to calculate IV rate of flow.

$$\begin{array}{ccccc} \textbf{Volume} & \times & \textbf{Calibration} & \times & \textbf{Time} & = & \textbf{Flow Rate} \\ \textbf{(ml / time)} & & \textbf{(gtts. / ml)} & & \textbf{(1 hr. / 60 min.)} & & \textbf{(gtts. / min.)} \end{array}$$

Example: Ordered: IV 5% D/W at 110 ml/hr.
Tubing drop factor: 15 gtts./ml
What is the rate of flow?

$$\frac{110 \text{ ml}}{1 \text{ hr.}} \times \frac{15 \text{ gtts.}}{1 \text{ ml}} \times \frac{1 \text{ hr.}}{60 \text{ min.}} = \frac{1650}{60} = 27.5 = 28 \text{ gtts./min.}$$

Problems to try. Answers to these problems appear at the end of 8.1 exercises.

a. Ordered: IV 5% D/W 100 ml/hr.
   Tubing calibration: 15 gtts./ml
   Rate of flow   _____

b.   Ordered: IV 0.45% Saline 125 ml/hr.
   Tubing drop factor: 20 gtts./ml
   Flow rate   _____

When the order is written for the volume to be given in a time period of more than one hour, you can use the formula method for determining rate of flow in one of two ways.

Example: Ordered: IV of 1000 ml to run in 8 hrs.
Drop factor: 20 gtts./ml
What is the flow rate?

One method is to divide total volume by total time to determine how many ml/hr.

$$\frac{1000 \text{ ml}}{8 \text{ hr}} = \frac{1000}{8} = 125 = 125 \text{ ml/hr.}$$

Then use the **Formula Method**.

$$\frac{125 \text{ ml} \times 20 \text{ gtts./ml}}{60 \text{ min.}} = \frac{2500}{60} = 41.6 = 42 \text{ gtts./min.}$$

Another method is to change the hours to minutes. (60 min. = 1 hr.)

$$8 \text{ hr.} \times 60 \text{ min.}/\text{hr.} = 8 \times 60 = 480 \text{ min.}$$

Then use the **Formula Method**.

$$\frac{100 \text{ ml} \times 20 \text{ gtts.}/\text{ml}}{480 \text{ min. (8 hrs.)}} = \frac{20000}{480} = 41.6 = 42 \text{ gtts.}/\text{min.}$$

Or use the **Factor-Label Method**.

$$\frac{10000 \text{ ml}}{8 \text{ hr.}} \times \frac{20 \text{ gtts.}}{\text{ml}} \times \frac{1 \text{ hr.}}{60 \text{ min.}} = 41.6 = 42 \text{ gtts.}/\text{min.}$$

Example: Ordered: IV of 3000 ml in 24 hrs.
Drop factor: 10 gtts./ml
What is the rate of flow?

Determine how many ml/hr.

$$\frac{3000 \text{ ml}}{24 \text{ hr.}} = \frac{3000}{24} = 125 = 125 \text{ ml}/\text{hr.}$$

Then use the **Formula Method**.

$$\frac{125 \text{ ml} \times 10 \text{ gtts.}/\text{ml}}{60 \text{ min.}} = \frac{1250}{60} = 20.8 = 21 \text{ gtts.}/\text{min.}$$

or

Convert 24 hours to minutes.

$$24 \text{ hrs.} \times 60 \text{ min.}/\text{hr.} = 1440 \text{ min.}$$

Then use the **Formula Method**.

$$\frac{3000 \text{ ml} \times 10 \text{ gtts.}/\text{ml}}{1440 \text{ min. (24 hrs.)}} = \frac{30000}{1440} = 20.8 = 21 \text{ gtts.}/\text{min.}$$

or

Use the **Factor-Label Method**.

$$\frac{3000 \text{ ml}}{24 \text{ hrs.}} \times \frac{10 \text{ gtts.}}{\text{ml}} \times \frac{1 \text{ hr.}}{60 \text{ min.}} = 20.8 = 21 \text{ gtts.}/\text{min.}$$

Problems to try.

c. Ordered: IV 2000 ml/24 hrs.
   Drop factor: 20 gtts./ml
   What is the flow rate?   _____

d. Ordered: IV 1000 ml/4 hrs.
   Drop factor: 15 gtts./ml
   What is the rate of flow?   _____

8.1   *Exercises*

Determine the rate of flow.

Ordered	Drop Factor	Rate of Flow
1. IV 5% D/W at 125 ml/hr.	15 gtts./ml	_____
2. IV 0.9% saline at 200 ml/hr.	15 gtts./ml	_____
3. IV 10% D/W at 100 ml/hr.	15 gtts./ml	_____
4. IV 5% D/W at 50 ml/hr.	15 gtts./ml	_____
5. IV 10% D/W at 100 ml/hr.	20 gtts./ml	_____
6. IV 0.9% saline at 200 ml/hr.	20 gtts./ml	_____

7. IV 5% D/W at 125 ml/hr.   20 gtts./ml   _____

8. IV to run 150 ml/hr.   15 gtts./ml   _____

9. IV 0.45% saline at 100 ml/hr.   60 gtts./ml   _____

10. IV lactated ringers at   60 gtts./ml   _____
      50 ml/hr.

11. IV of 1000 ml in 8 hrs.   15 gtts./ml   _____

12. IV of 3000 ml in 24 hrs.   20 gtts./ml   _____

13. IV of 2000 ml in 8 hrs.   15 gtts./ml   _____

14. IV of 500 ml in 6 hrs.   20 gtts./ml   _____

15. IV of 250 ml in 4 hrs.   60 gtts./ml   _____

16. IV of 500 ml in 6 hrs.   60 gtts./ml   _____

17. IV of 1000 ml in 8 hrs.   60 gtts./ml   _____

18. IV of 1000 ml in 10 hrs.   20 gtts./ml   _____

19. IV of 1000 ml in 12 hrs.   15 gtts./ml   _____

20. IV of 250 ml in 2 hrs.   15 gtts./ml   _____

Answers to Problems to try.

a. 25 gtts./min.   b. 42 gtts./min.   c. 28 gtts./min.   d. 62 or 63 gtts./min.

Space Provided for Student Work

8.2 Rate of Flow—Division Factor Method

The division factor method can be used to determine flow rate. **It can only be used if the volume to be given is expressed in ml/hr. (ml/60 min.)**. Because you are restricting the time to 60 min., the drop factor can be divided into 60 to obtain a constant number. This number is called the division factor. You can obtain the division factor for any IV administration set by dividing the drop factor of the set into 60.

Division Factor Method
To calculate the rate of flow you need the following information:

    a. the total volume of fluid to be infused in ml;
    b. the division factor (60 ÷ drop factor).

$$\frac{\text{Volume (ml)}}{\text{Division Factor}} = \textbf{Rate of Flow (gtts./ min.)}$$

Example: Ordered: IV at 100 ml/hr.
                   Drop factor: 15 gtts./ml

               60 min. ÷ 15 gtts./ml = 4   calculate the division factor

               $\frac{100 \text{ ml}}{4}$ = 25 gtts./min.   use the **Division Factor Method**

Example: Ordered: IV 100 ml/hr.
                   Drop factor: 10 gtts./ml

               60 min. ÷ 10 gtts./ml = 6   calculate the division factor

               $\frac{100 \text{ ml}}{6}$ = 16.6 = 17 gtts./min.   use the **Division Factor Method**

Example: Ordered: IV 75 ml/hr.
                   Drop factor: 60 gtts./ml

               60 min. ÷ 60 gtts./ml = 1   calculate the division factor

               $\frac{75 \text{ ml}}{1}$ = 75 gtts./min.   use the **Division Factor Method**

Note: In the previous example, when a micro drip set is used and calibrated at 60 gtts./min, the division factor is one (1). The flow rate is the same as the volume in ml/hr.

The following table shows the division factors for various tubing calibrations.

Drop Factor	**Division Factor**
10 gtts./ml	**6 (60 ÷ 10)**
15 gtts./ml	**4 (60 ÷ 15)**
20 gtts./ml	**3 (60 ÷ 20)**
60 gtts./ml	**1 (60 ÷ 60)**

Problems to try. Answers to these problems appear at the end of 8.2 exercises.

a. Ordered: IV rate at 200 ml/hr.
   Drop factor: 15 gtts./ml
   What is the flow rate? _____

b. Ordered: IV 100 ml/hr.
   Drop factor: 60 gtts./ml
   What is the flow rate? _____

8.2 *Exercises*

Determine the rate of flow.

Ordered	Drop Factor	Rate of Flow
1. IV 50 ml/hr.	60 gtts./ml	_____
2. IV 125 ml/hr.	20 gtts./ml	_____

3. IV 100 ml/hr.   20 gtts./ml   _____

4. IV 125 ml/hr.   15 gtts./ml   _____

5. IV 75 ml/hr.   20 gtts./ml   _____

6. IV 100 ml/hr.   15 gtts./ml   _____

7. IV 150 ml/hr.   10 gtts./ml   _____

8. IV 200 ml/hr.   20 gtts./ml   _____

9. IV 50 ml/hr.   20 gtts./ml   _____

10. IV 150 ml/hr.   20 gtts./ml   _____

11. IV 200 ml/hr.   10 gtts./ml   _____

12. IV 200 ml/hr.   15 gtts./ml   _____

13. IV 50 ml/hr.   15 gtts./ml   _____

14. IV 100 ml/hr.   10 gtts./ml   _____

15. IV 150 ml/hr   15 gtts./ml   _____

Answers to Problems to try.

a. 50 gtts./min.   b. 100 gtts./min.

Space Provided for Student Work

8.3   Total Time

You may need to calculate the total time an IV is to run. The formula method can be adjusted to give a formula that will calculate the total time.

$$\frac{\text{Volume (ml)} \times \text{Calibration (gtts./ml)}}{\text{Rate of flow (gtts./min.)}} = \textbf{Total time in minutes}$$

or

$$\underset{\text{(ml)}}{\textbf{Volume}} \times \underset{\text{(gtts./ml)}}{\textbf{Calibration}} \times \underset{\text{(1 min./gtts.)}}{\textbf{Inverted Rate of Flow}} = \textbf{Total time in min.}$$

Example: Ordered: 1500 ml IV
Drop factor: 10 gtts./ml
Rate of flow: 50 gtts./min.
How long will the IV run?

$$\frac{1500 \text{ ml} \times 10 \text{ gtts./ml}}{50 \text{ gtts./min.}}$$ substitute information into the formula

$$\frac{1500 \times 10}{50} = \frac{15000}{50}$$ do the multiplication first

$$15000 \div 50 = 300 \text{ min.}$$ divide and label your answer

It is inappropriate to say that an IV will run 300 min. Convert the minutes to hours by dividing by 60 (60 min. = 1 hr.)

$$\frac{300}{60} = 5 \text{ hours}$$

or

Factor Label Method

$$\frac{1500 \text{ ml}}{1} \times \frac{10 \text{ gtts.}}{1 \text{ ml}} \times \frac{1 \text{ min.}}{50 \text{ gtts.}} = 300 \text{ min.} = 5 \text{ hr.}$$

Example: Ordered: 1000 ml IV
Drop factor: 20 gtts./ml
Rate of flow: 42 gtts./min.
How long will the IV run?

$$\frac{1000 \text{ ml} \times 20 \text{ gtts./ml}}{42 \text{ gtts./min.}} = \frac{20000}{42} = 476.19 = 476 \text{ min. (round)}$$

$$\frac{476}{60} = 7.93 = 8 \text{ hours} \qquad \text{round to the nearest half hour}$$

or

Factor Label Method

$$\frac{1000 \text{ ml}}{1} \times \frac{20 \text{ gtts.}}{\text{ml}} \times \frac{1 \text{ min.}}{42 \text{ gtts.}} = 476 \text{ min.} = 8 \text{ hr.}$$

Problems to try. Answers to these problems appear at the end of 8.3 exercises.

a.   Ordered: 1200 ml IV
Drop factor: 15 gtts./ml
Rate of flow: 50 gtts./min.
How long will the IV run?   _____

b.   Ordered: 2000 ml IV
Drop factor: 20 gtts./ml
Rate of flow: 60 gtts./min.
How long will the IV run?   _____

Space Provided for Student Work

8.3 Exercises

	Ordered	Drop Factor	Rate of Flow	Total Time	
				Minutes	Hours
1.	2000 ml	15 gtts./ml	50 gtts./min.	_____	_____
2.	1000 ml	20 gtts./ml	50 gtts./min.	_____	_____
3.	1000 ml	15 gtts./ml	31 gtts./min.	_____	_____
4.	3000 ml	20 gtts./ml	42 gtts./min.	_____	_____
5.	250 ml	60 gtts./ml	63 gtts./min.	_____	_____
6.	1000 ml	20 gtts./ml	33 gtts./min.	_____	_____
7.	250 ml	15 gtts./ml	31 gtts./min.	_____	_____
8.	2000 ml	15 gtts./ml	63 gtts./min.	_____	_____
9.	500 ml	20 gtts./ml	28 gtts./min.	_____	_____
10.	500 ml	60 gtts./ml	84 gtts./min.	_____	_____

Answers to Problems to try.

a. 6 hrs. b. 11 hrs.

8.4   Pediatric IVs

Children receiving IV solutions may get them on either a continuous or intermittent basis.

Electronic delivery devices are usually utilized for pediatric patients because of the small volumes of fluid and/or medication given to the patients.

Intermittent medication dosages are frequently given with a special IV set designed to deliver small, accurate amounts of IV fluids. These sets are calibrated in 1 ml increments, so exact measurement is possible. These sets are all micro-drop sets and are calibrated to deliver 60 gtts./ml. They are known by the trade names Buretrol, Soluset, and Volutrol.

When giving medication through these sets, a flush, usually 15 ml or 20 ml, is given after the medication to ensure the delivery of all the medication to the patient. This would not apply to infants or children who are receiving very small amounts of fluid.

To calculate the flow rate, the amount of solution in the flush should be added to the medication amount.

Note: When administering the medication, the flush is always given separately.

The calculation of flow rates may be done using either the **Formula Method** or the **Division Factor Method**. You can only use the division factor method if the volume to be given is expressed in ml/hr.

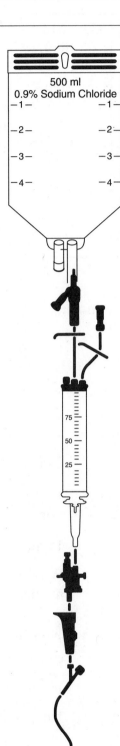

> **TO CALCULATE THE FLOW RATE OF A PEDIATRIC IV:**
>   **Step 1.** Read the medication label to determine what volume contains the correct dosage.
>   **Step 2.** Determine the amount of IV fluid to be added to the medication.
>   (diluted volume—medication volume = IV solution volume)
>   **Step 3.** Add total diluted volume and flush volume
>   (diluted volume + flush volume = total infusion volume)
>   **Step 4.** Calculate rate of flow using the formula method.
>
> $$\frac{\text{total infusion volume} \times \text{drop factor}}{\text{time (min.)}} = \text{flow rate}$$

Example: An antibiotic dosage of 50 mg has been ordered diluted in 15 ml of 5% D/W to infuse over 20 min. A 15 ml flush of 5% D/W is to follow. The label reads 50 mg/2 ml. Calculate the amount of IV fluid needed to mix the medication and the flow rate for administration.

Step 1.   Read the medication label to determine what volume contains 50 mg.

2 ml contains 50 mg

Step 2.   Determine the amount of IV fluid needed to dilute the 2 ml of medication to yield a 15 ml infusion.

15 ml − 2 ml = 13 ml

When putting the solution in the Buretrol you would use 2 ml of medication plus 13 ml of IV fluid for a total of 15 ml.

Step 3.   Add the infusion volume to the flush volume. **This step is only done for calculation of the flow rate not for administration.**

15 ml + 15 ml = 30 ml   total infusion volume

Step 4.   Determine the rate of flow.

$$\frac{30 \text{ ml} \times 60 \text{ gtts./ml}}{20 \text{ min.}} = 90 \text{ gtts./min.}$$

Example: An antibiotic dosage of 75 mg has been ordered diluted to 15 ml to infuse in 30 minutes. A 15 ml flush is to follow. The label reads 75 mg/2 ml. Calculate the amount of IV fluid needed to mix the medication and the flow rate for administration.

Step 1.   Read the medication label to determine what volume contains 75 mg.

2 ml contains 75 mg

Step 2.   Determine the amount of IV fluid needed to dilute the 2 ml of medication to yield a 15 ml infusion.

15 ml − 2 ml = 13 ml

When putting the solution in the Buretrol you would use 2 ml of medication plus 13 ml of IV fluid for a total of 15 ml.

Step 3.   Add the infusion volume to the flush volume. **This step is only done for calculation of the flow rate not for administration**.

15 ml + 15 ml = 30 ml   total infusion volume

Step 4.   Determine the rate of flow.

$$\frac{30 \text{ ml} \times 60 \text{ gtts./ml}}{30 \text{ min.}} = 60 \text{ gtts./min.}$$

Problems to try. Answers to these problems appear at the end of 8.4 exercises.

a. Medication of 50 mg is ordered diluted to 50 ml. Infuse over 30 minutes and follow with a 15 ml flush. The label reads 25 mg/ml. Calculate the amount of IV fluid needed to mix the medication and the flow rate for administration.

b. IV medication of 160 mg is ordered. The label reads 40 mg/ml. Dilute to 50 ml and infuse over 45 min. Follow with a 15 ml flush. Calculate the amount of IV fluid needed to mix the medication and the flow rate for administration.

8.4   Exercises

---

a. Determine the amount of IV solution needed to mix the following medications; and b. calculate the flow rate for administration. All tubing is calibrated at 60 gtts./ml.

1. IV medication of 50 mg is ordered diluted to 50 ml. Infuse over 45 min. with a 15 ml flush to follow. The label reads 50 mg/3 ml.

    a. _____

    b. _____

2. IV medication of 100 mg is ordered diluted to 50 ml. Infuse over 30 min. and follow with a 15 ml flush. The label reads 100 mg/2 ml.

    a. _____

    b. _____

3. IV medication of 20 mg is ordered diluted to 15 ml. Infuse over 30 min. and follow with a 15 ml flush. The label reads 20 mg/ml.

    a. _____

    b. _____

4. IV medication of 750 mg is ordered diluted to 20 ml. Infuse over 40 min. and follow with a 15 ml flush. The label reads 750 mg/ml.

    a. _____

    b. _____

5. IV medication of 1.5 g is ordered diluted to 30 ml. Infuse over 40 min. and follow with a 15 ml flush. The label reads 1.5 g/3 ml

    a. _____

    b. _____

6. IV medication of 200 mg is ordered diluted to 40 ml. Infuse over 40 min. and follow with a 15 ml flush. The label reads 100 mg/2.5 ml.

    a. _____

    b. _____

7. IV medication of 80 mg is ordered diluted to 80 ml. Infuse over 60 min. and follow with a 15 ml flush. The label reads 40 mg/ml.

    a. _____

    b. _____

8. IV medication of 5 mg is ordered diluted to 10 ml. Infuse over 10 min. and follow with a 15 ml flush. The label reads 2.5 mg/ml.

    a. _____

    b. _____

9. IV medication of 100 mg is ordered diluted to 20 ml. Infuse over 15 min. and follow with a 15 ml flush. The label reads 50 mg/ml.

    a. _____

    b. _____

10. IV medication of 0.5 g is ordered diluted to 40 ml. Infuse over 45 min. and follow with a 15 ml flush. The label reads 0.5 g/2 ml.

a. _____

b. _____

Answers to Problems to try.

a. 48 ml, 130 gtts./min.   b. 46 ml, 87 gtts./min.

_____

Space Provided for Student Work

_____

8.5 Piggyback IV Solutions

IV medications are frequently ordered to run piggyback with IV fluids. Usually the medication is dissolved in 50 to 100 ml of solution and runs for a specific period of time.

When the piggyback is running, the main IV bag is either clamped shut or hung lower than the piggyback to allow the secondary fluid to infuse.

Between piggybacks, the vein is kept open by running the IV solution.

To control the total volume of IV fluid, the piggyback medication must be included in the total IV fluid volume. The total time the IV is to run includes the time for all piggybacks.

The rate of flow for the piggyback and the IV between piggybacks is calculated using the Formula Method.

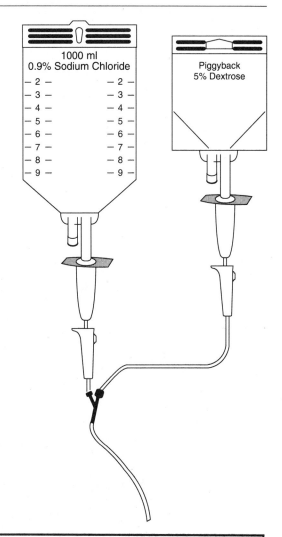

TO CALCULATE RATE OF FLOW FOR THE PIGGYBACK AND THE IV BETWEEN PIGGYBACKS:

Step 1. Calculate the rate of flow for each piggyback.

Step 2. Calculate the number of piggybacks to be given.

Step 3. Determine the total time and total fluid volume for all piggybacks.
(number of piggybacks) × (time for each piggyback)
(number of piggybacks) × (volume for each piggyback)

Step 4. Determine the amount of time and volume of fluid remaining.
(total time) − (total time for piggybacks)
(total volume) − (total volume for piggybacks)

Step 5. Calculate the rate of flow of the IV between piggybacks, using the amounts from step 4.

Example: The patient is to receive 2000 ml of IV fluids in 24 hr. Also ordered is a piggyback medication dissolved in 100 ml of fluid to run for 30 minutes. The piggyback is to be given every 8 hours. The IV is to be kept open between piggybacks with 5% D/W. The drop factor on all tubing is 15 gtts./ml.

What is the rate of flow for each piggyback?
What is the rate of flow for the IV between piggybacks?

Step 1.   Calculate the rate of flow for each piggyback.

$$\frac{100 \times 15}{30} = 50 \text{ gtts./min.}$$

Step 2.   Calculate the number of piggybacks to be given in 24 hours.

$24 \div 8 = 3$ piggybacks

Step 3.   Determine the total time in minutes used for all piggybacks.

3×30 min. $= 90$ min.

Determine the total fluid volume for all piggybacks.

3×100 ml $= 300$ ml

Step 4.   Determine the amount of time in minutes remaining.

24 hr = 1440 min. $1440 - 90 = 1350$ min.

Determine the volume of IV fluid remaining.

2000 ml $-$ 300 ml $=$ 1700 ml

Step 5.   Calculate the rate of flow of the IV between piggybacks, using the amounts from Step 4.

$$\frac{1700 \times 15}{1350} = 18.9 = 19 \text{ gtt./min.}$$

Example: The patient is to receive 1000 ml IV fluids every 12 hours. In addition, ordered is a piggyback medication dissolved in 100 ml of solution to run for 30 minutes. The piggyback is ordered q.6h. The IV is to be kept open between piggybacks. The drop factor on all tubing is 20 gtts./ml.

What is the rate of flow for each piggyback?
What is the rate of flow for the IV between piggybacks?

Step 1.   Calculate the rate of flow for each piggyback.

$$\frac{100 \times 20}{30} = 66.7 = 67 \text{ gtts./min.}$$

Step 2.   Calculate the number of piggybacks to be given in 12 hours.

$12 \div 6 = 2$ piggybacks

Step 3.   Determine the total time in minutes used for all piggybacks.

2×30 min. $= 60$ min.

Determine the total fluid volume for all piggybacks.

2×100 ml $= 200$ ml

Step 4.   Determine the amount of time in minutes remaining.

12 hr $= 720$ min. $720 - 60 = 660$ min.

Determine the volume of IV fluid remaining.

1000 ml $- 200$ ml $= 800$ ml

Step 5.   Calculate the rate of flow of the IV between piggybacks, using the amounts from Step 4.

$$\frac{800 \times 20}{660} = 24.2 = 24 \text{ gtts./min.}$$

Problems to try. Answers to these problems appear at the end of 8.5 exercises.

a. The patient is to receive 3000 ml IV fluids every 24 hours. In addition, ordered is a piggyback medication dissolved in 100 ml of solution to run for 30 minutes. The piggyback is ordered q.12h. The IV is to be kept open between piggybacks. The drop factor on all tubing is 15 gtts./ml.

What is the rate of flow for each piggyback?   _____

What is the rate of flow for the IV between piggybacks?   _____

b. Ordered: 2000 ml IV fluids in 12 hours
Piggyback medication in 50 ml to run 30 min. q.12h.
Drop factor for all tubing is 20 gtts./ml

What is the rate of flow for each piggyback?   _____

What is the rate of flow for the IV between piggybacks?   _____

c. Ordered: 1500 ml IV fluids in 24 hours
Piggyback medication in 75 ml to run 30 min. q.8h.
Drop factor for all tubing is 15 gtts./ml

What is the rate of flow for each piggyback? _____

What is the rate of flow for the IV between piggybacks? _____

8.5 Exercises

---

1. Ordered: 2000 ml IV fluids in 24 hours
Piggyback medication in 100 ml to run 30 min. q.8h.
Drop factor for all tubing is 20 gtts./ml

What is the rate of flow for each piggyback? _____

What is the rate of flow for the IV between piggybacks? _____

2. Ordered: 3000 ml IV fluids in 24 hours
Piggyback medication in 50 ml to run 30 min. q.6h.
Drop factor for all tubing is 15 gtts./ml

What is the rate of flow for each piggyback? _____

What is the rate of flow for the IV between piggybacks? _____

3. Ordered: 1500 ml IV fluids in 12 hours
Piggyback medication in 50 ml to run 1 hr. q.6h.
Drop factor for all tubing is 15 gtts./ml

What is the rate of flow for each piggyback? _____

What is the rate of flow for the IV between piggybacks? _____

4.   Ordered: 1800 ml IV fluids in 24 hours
Piggyback medication in 100 ml to run 60 min. q.6h.
Drop factor for all tubing is 20 gtts./ml

What is the rate of flow for each piggyback?   _____

What is the rate of flow for the IV between piggybacks?   _____

5.   Ordered: 2000 ml IV fluids in 24 hours
Piggyback medication in 50 ml to run 30 min. q.8h.
Drop factor for all tubing is 15 gtts./ml

What is the rate of flow for each piggyback?   _____

What is the rate of flow for the IV between piggybacks?   _____

6.   Ordered: 1500 ml IV fluids in 12 hours
Piggyback medication in 100 ml to run 60 min. q.6h.
Drop factor for all tubing is 15 gtts./ml

What is the rate of flow for each piggyback?   _____

What is the rate of flow for the IV between piggybacks?   _____

7.   Ordered: 2000 ml IV fluids in 24 hours
Piggyback medication in 100 ml to run 60 min. q.6h.
Drop factor for all tubing is 20 gtts./ml

What is the rate of flow for each piggyback?   _____

What is the rate of flow for the IV between piggybacks?   _____

8. Ordered: 2000 ml IV fluids in 12 hours
    Piggyback medication in 75 ml to run 60 min. q.12h.
    Drop factor for all tubing is 20 gtts./ml

    What is the rate of flow for each piggyback? _____

    What is the rate of flow for the IV between piggybacks? _____

9. Ordered: 1000 ml IV fluids in 8 hours
    Piggyback medication in 50 ml to run 30 min. q.4h.
    Drop factor for all tubing is 20 gtts./ml

    What is the rate of flow for each piggyback? _____

    What is the rate of flow for the IV between piggybacks? _____

10. Ordered: 1500 ml IV fluids in 8 hours
    Piggyback medication in 50 ml to run 30 min. q.4h.
    Drop factor for all tubing is 15 gtts./ml

    What is the rate of flow for each piggyback? _____

    What is the rate of flow for the IV between piggybacks? _____

Answers to Problems to try.

a. 50 gtts./min.; 30 gtts./min.   b. 33 gtts./min.; 57 gtts./min.
c. 38 gtts./min.; 14 gtts./min.

8.6   *Drug Infusion Rate of Flow*

Many critical care medications are added to the IV solution and infused at the rate of a specified concentration of medication per unit of time. This is called drug infusion rate, and is expressed in ml/min. or ml/hr.

Because of the exact amounts needed, these solutions are administered via an IV infusion pump (see p. 252). The drug infusion rate is calculated and programmed into the pump. If a pump is not available, mini- or micro-drip tubing should be used and closely monitored.

TO CALCULATE THE DRUG INFUSION RATE:
   a. **determine the solution strength;**
   b. **determine what has been ordered;**
   c. **using one of the four methods for calculating patient dosage (see 7.2), calculate the drug infusion rate in ml/min.;**
   d. **calculate drug infusion rate in ml/hr. (ml/min.× 60 min.)**

Example: Order: LIDOCAINE® 2 g IV in 500 ml 5% D/W to run at 2 mg/min. Calculate the drug infusion rate in ml/min. and ml/hr.

What is the solution strength of the medication? (2 g/500 ml)
What dosage has been ordered? (2 mg/min.)
Calculate the drug infusion rate in ml/min.

1. **Dosage Formula**

$$2 \text{ mg/min.} \div \frac{2 \text{ g}}{500 \text{ ml}} = \qquad \text{Remember to change g to mg.}$$

$$2 \text{ mg/min.} \times \frac{500 \text{ ml}}{2000 \text{ mg}} = \frac{1000}{2000} = 0.5 \text{ ml/min.}$$

2. **DQA Proportion**

$$\frac{2 \text{ mg/min.}}{2000 \text{ mg}} = \frac{X \text{ ml/min.}}{500 \text{ ml}}$$

$$1000 = 2000 \, X$$

$$\frac{1000}{2000} = 0.5 \text{ ml/min.}$$

3. **DHQ Formula**

$$\frac{2 \text{ mg/min.}}{2000 \text{ mg}} \times 500 \text{ ml} = \frac{1000}{2000} = 0.5 \text{ ml/min.}$$

4. **Label Proportion**

$$\frac{2000 \text{ mg}}{500 \text{ ml}} = \frac{2 \text{ mg/min.}}{X \text{ ml/min.}}$$

$$2000 \text{ X} = 1000$$

$$X = \frac{1000}{2000} = 0.5 \text{ ml/min.}$$

Calculate the drug infusion rate in ml/hr., by multiplying the ml/min. by 60 min./hr.

$$0.5 \text{ ml/min.} \times 60 \text{ min./hr.} = 30 \text{ ml/hr.}$$

This calculation allows you to estimate when to order the next bag of medication.

Example: Order: heparin 20,000 U IV in 500 ml NS to run at 1200 U/hr.
Calculate the drug infusion rate in ml/min. and ml/hr.

What is the solution strength of the medication? (20000 U/500 ml)
What dosage has been ordered? (1200 U/hr.)
Calculate the drug infusion rate in ml/min.

1. **Dosage Formula**

$$1200 \text{ U/hr.} \div \frac{20000 \text{ U}}{500 \text{ ml}} =$$

$$1200 \text{ U/hr.} \times \frac{500 \text{ ml}}{20000 \text{ U}} = \frac{600000}{20000} = 30 \text{ ml/hr.}$$

2. **DQA Proportion**

$$\frac{1200 \text{ U/hr.}}{20000 \text{ U}} = \frac{X \text{ ml/hr.}}{500 \text{ ml}}$$

$$600000 = 20000 \text{ X}$$

$$\frac{600000}{20000} = 30 \text{ ml/hr.}$$

3. **DHQ Formula**

$$\frac{1200 \text{ U/hr.}}{20000 \text{ U}} \times 500 \text{ ml} = \frac{600000}{20000} = 30 \text{ ml/hr.}$$

4. **Label Proportion**

$$\frac{20000 \text{ U}}{500 \text{ ml}} = \frac{1200 \text{ U/hr.}}{X \text{ ml/hr.}}$$

$$20000 \text{ X} = 600000$$

$$X = \frac{600000}{20000} = 30 \text{ ml/hr.}$$

Calculate the drug infusion rate in ml/min. by dividing the ml/hr. by 60 min./hr.

$$30 \text{ ml/hr.} \div 60 \text{ min./hr.} = 0.5 \text{ ml/min.}$$

When necessary round ml/min. to hundredths and ml/hr. to the nearest whole milliliter.

Problems to try. Answers to these problems appear at the end of 8.6 exercises.

a. Order: ISUPREL® (isoproterenol hydrochloride) 2 mg IV in 500 ml 5% D/W to run at 5 μg/min. Calculate the drug infusion rate in ml/min. and ml/hr.

b. Order: LIDOCAINE® 2 g IV in 1000 ml 5% D/W to run at 3 mg/min. Calculate the drug infusion rate in ml/min. and ml/hr.

c. Order: DOPAMINE® 800 mg IV in 500 ml 5% D/W to run at 40 mg/hr. Calculate the drug infusion rate in ml/min. and ml/hr.

8.6 Exercises

Calculate the drug infusion rate in ml/min. and ml/hr.

1. Order: PRONESTYL® (procainamide hydrochloride) 0.5 g IV in 250 ml 5% D/W to run at 2 mg/min.

2. Order: LIDOCAINE® 2 g IV in 1000 ml 5% D/W to run at 4 mg/min.

3. Order: LIDOCAINE® 1 g IV in 250 ml 5% D/W to run at 2 mg/min.

4. Order: Heparin 20,000 U IV in 1000 ml 5% D/W to run at 1400 U/hr

5. Order: Heparin 10,000 U IV in 100 ml 5% D/W to run at 1200 U/hr.

6. Order: LIDOCAINE® 2 g IV in 500 ml 5% D/W to run at 4 mg/min.

7. Order: Heparin 40,000 U IV in 1000 ml 5% D/W to run at 1200 U/hr.

8. Order: DOPAMINE® 400 mg IV in 500 ml 5% D/W to run at 400 μg/min.

9. Order: ISUPREL® (isoproterenol hydrochloride) 2 mg IV in 500 ml 5% D/W to run at 3 μg/min.

10. Order: Heparin 20,000 units IV in 1000 ml 5% D/W to run at 1600 U/hr.

Answers to Problems to try.

a. 1.25 ml/min.;   75 ml/hr.   b. 1.5 ml/min.;   90 ml/hr.   c. 0.42 ml/min.;   25 ml/hr.

_____

Space Provided for Student Work

_____

8.7   Monitoring Flow Rates

Some IVs are administered by using the gravity flow method. The rate is regulated by a roller clamp on the tubing, and the drops are counted as they fall into the drip chamber.

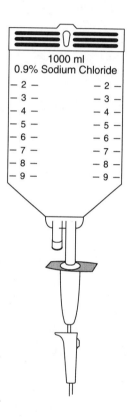

Electronic regulators are used extensively for safety and for more efficient control of infusions. They are set to deliver a specific flow rate and are equipped with alarms to alert personnel if the rate is not maintained. There are two types in use: controllers and pumps, which are pictured on the next page.

Controllers
Controllers work in the same way as a gravity IV. The rate of flow is regulated by the controller pinching the IV tube.

Pumps
Pumps physically pump the fluid into the patient.

(Courtesy Abbott Laboratories)

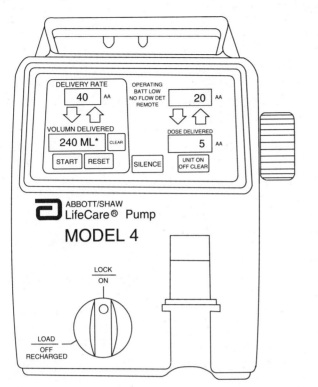

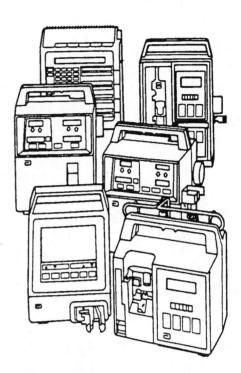

Chapter 8   Test

Calculate the rate of flow for the following.

1. Ordered: IV fluid of 0.9% saline to run at 125 ml/hr.
    Drop factor: 15 gtts./ml

    Flow rate   _____

2. Ordered: IV fluid of 5% D/W to run at 50 ml/hr.
    Drop factor: 60 gtts./ml

    Flow rate   _____

3. Ordered: IV fluid of lactated ringers 1000 ml to run for 10 hr.
    Drop factor: 15 gtts./ml

    Flow rate   _____

4. Ordered: 1000 ml of IV fluid to run for 12 hr.
    Drop factor: 20 gtts./ml

    Flow rate   _____

5. Ordered: 3000 ml of IV fluid to run for 24 hr.
    Drop factor: 10 gtts./ml

    Flow rate   _____

6. Ordered: 1000 ml 5% D/W q.8h.
    Drop factor: 15 gtts./ml

    Flow rate   _____

7. Ordered: 1000 ml lactated ringers q.12h.
    Drop factor: 15 gtts./ml

    Flow rate _____

Calculate: a. the amount of IV fluid needed to mix the medication, and b. the flow rate for administration. All tubing is calibrated at 60 gtts./ml.

8. Ordered: IV medication of 100 mg diluted to 30 ml. The label reads 50 mg/ml. Infuse over 30 min. and follow with a 15 ml flush.

    a. _____

    b. _____

9. Ordered: IV medication of 20 mg diluted to 30 ml. Infuse over 30 min. and follow with a 20 ml flush. The label reads 5 mg/ml.

    a. _____

    b. _____

10. Ordered: IV antibiotic of 500 mg diluted to 20 ml. The label reads 500 mg/5 ml. Infuse over 20 min. and follow with a 20 ml flush.

    a. _____

    b. _____

11. Ordered: IV medication of 1 gram diluted to 50 ml. The label reads 500 mg/3 ml. Infuse over 45 min. and follow with a 15 ml flush.

    a. _____

    b   _____

12.   Ordered: IV medication of 250 mg diluted to 75 ml. The label reads 125 mg/ml. Infuse over one hour and follow with a 15 ml flush.

a.   _____

b.   _____

13.   Ordered: IV medication of 500 mg diluted to 50 ml. The label reads 200 mg/ml. Infuse over 45 min. and follow with a 20 ml flush.

a.   _____

b.   _____

Calculate the total time the IV is to run.

14.   Ordered: 1000 ml IV
      Drop factor: 15 gtts./ml
      Rate of flow: 42 gtts./min.

      How long will the IV run?   _____

15.   Ordered: 1500 ml IV
      Drop factor: 20 gtts./ml
      Rate of flow: 31 gtts./min.

      How long will the IV run?   _____

16.   Ordered: 500 ml IV
      Drop factor: 60 gtts./ml
      Rate of flow: 50 gtts./min.

      How long will the IV run?   _____

17.   Ordered: 250 ml IV
      Drop factor: 60 gtts./ml
      Rate of flow: 20 gtts./min.

      How long will the IV run?   _____

Calculate: a. the rate of flow for piggyback medications, and b. the rate of flow
for the IV between piggybacks.

18.   Ordered: 2000 ml IV fluids in 12 hours
      Piggyback medication in 60 ml to run 60 min. q.6h.
      Drop factor for all tubing is 15 gtts./ml

      a.   _____

      b.   _____

19.   Ordered: 1000 ml IV fluids in 8 hours
      Piggyback medication in 75 ml to run 30 min. q.4h.
      Drop factor for all tubing is 20 gtts./ml

      a.   _____

      b.   _____

20.   Ordered: 1000 ml IV fluids in 12 hours
      Piggyback medication in 50 ml to run 30 min. g.4h.
      Drop factor for all tubing is 15 gtts./ml

      a.   _____

      b.   _____

21. Ordered: 3000 ml IV fluids in 24 hours
     Piggyback medication in 50 ml to run 30 min. q.12h.
     Drop factor for all tubing is 20 gtts./ml

     a. _____

     b. _____

22. Ordered: 1500 ml IV fluids in 8 hours
     Piggyback medication in 75 ml to run 45 min. q.4h.
     Drop factor for all tubing is 15 gtts./ml

     a. _____

     b. _____

23. Ordered: 3000 ml IV fluids in 24 hours
     Piggyback medication in 100 ml to run 1 hr. q.8h.
     Drop factor for all tubing is 15 gtts./ml

     a. _____

     b. _____

24. Ordered: 500 ml IV fluids in 8 hours
     Piggyback medication in 50 ml to run 30 min. q.4h.
     Drop factor for all tubing is 60 gtts./ml

     a. _____

     b. _____

25. Ordered: 500 ml IV fluids in 12 hours
     Piggyback medication in 75 ml to run 1 hr. q.6h.
     Drop factor for all tubing is 60 gtts./ml

     a. _____

     b. _____

Calculate the drug infusion rate for the following in ml/min. and ml/hr.

26. Order: LIDOCAINE® 2 g IV in 500 ml 5% D/W to run at 3 mg/min.

27. Order: ISUPREL® (isoproterenol hydrochloride) 4 mg IV in 100 ml 5% D/W to run at 3 μg/min.

28. Order: nitroglycerin 8 mg IV in 500 ml 5% D/W to run at 5 μg/min.

29. Order: Heparin 20,000 U IV in 500 ml 5% D/W to run at 1200 U/hr.

Space Provided for Student Work

Appendix A

A Brief History of Measurement

Our records of measurement date back to about 6000 B.C. from civilizations along the Nile. Early dimensions were based on parts of the body. The pyramids were built 500 cubits on a side; Noah built the ark $50 \times 100 \times 150$ cubits. Most measurements were in multiples or parts of a cubit. For example,

cubit	elbow to tip of middle finger
span	width of open hand fingertip to fingertip; 2 spans = 1 cubit
palm	width across hand; 3 palms = 1 span
hand	length of hand; now standardized to $4\frac{1}{2}$ inches
yard	gird, a man's belt; or, King Henry's nose to thumb with arm outstretched
fathom	length from fingertip to fingertip with arms outstretched
inch	length across thumb; or width of fingerjoints
rod	length of 16 men standing heel to toe
foot	$\frac{1}{16}$ of a rod
pace	one walking step in Germany; two walking steps in Rome
mile	1000 paces
acre	amount of land that a yoke of oxen could plow in a day
furlong	length of furrow across a square 10-acre field
knot	about 1000 fathoms; a sea mile

In 1324, King Edward II decreed that the official *inch* was equal to "three barleycorns, round and dried, from the midst of the ear, laid end to end." In 1496, King Henry I decreed the *yard* as the distance from the tip of his nose to the end of his thumb, arm outstretched. In medieval Germany, the length of the *rute*, or *rod*, was established by the "first 16 men leaving church on Sunday morning standing heel to toe." The overall length was the right and lawful *rod*, and one-sixteenth of the rod was the right and lawful *foot*. The Roman legionnaires strode out a *mile*; their mile was 1000 paces or about 1618 yards. The British changed this to 1760 yards, but in many European countries, the mile is smaller or, in some cases, larger than the British mile.

In addition to length units, there were early standards of weight and volume. In Genesis 23:16, we read that Abraham "bought a burial field for 400 shekel-weight of silver." In 1215, the Magna Carta established the "London quart" as the primary unit of volume.

Each country introduced its own standards, and there was often no relationship between them. Even today, the English or Customary system of measurement contains 85 different units, some of which are defined to measure particular objects. For example,

fortnight	14 days, and 14 nights
carat	equivalent weight of a carob seed; used to measure gold
square	10×10 or 100 square feet of roofing material
bolt	120 linear feet of fabric
load	1 cubic yard of gravel
Firkin	56 pounds of lard
vara	land measure; $33\frac{1}{3}$ inches in Texas; 33 inches in California; 32 inches in Spain; 43 inches in Latin America
skein	360 linear feet of yarn
catty	$1\frac{1}{3}$ pounds of tea
cord	128 cubic feet of wood ($4 \times 4 \times 8$ feet)

Moreover, the conversion numbers between bushel and peck, grains and ounce, square feet and acre, feet and mile, pint and gallon, etc. are hard to remember. In the English system there are two kings of pounds, miles, and quarts, eight kinds of tons, and 58 different sizes of bushels? A bushel =

60 lb. avoirdupois	45 lb. apples	64 lb. plums
47 lb. barley	60 lb. beans	48 lb. quinces
56 lb. beets	20 lb. bran	60 lb. rutabaga
48 lb. buckwheat	50 lb. cabbage	60 lb. rye-meal
50 lb. carrots	100 lb. cement	62 lb. ground salt
20 lb. charcoal	40 lb. coke	85 lb. coarse salt
75 lb. coal	56 lb. cherries	45 lb. Timothy seed
56 lb corn	60 lb. corn in Indiana	60 lb. turnips
40 lb. cranberries	60 lb. clover seeds	60 lb. wheat
50 lb. chestnuts	50 lb. cornmeal	45 lb. rice
40 lb. currents	50 lb. cucumbers	56 lb. rye
14 lb. grass seed	48 lb. grapes	100 lb. sand
80 lb. lime	60 lb. hominy	60 lb. tomatoes
55 lb. onion	48 lb. peaches	50 lb. walnuts
32 lb. oats in NJ	28 lb. oats in CT	60 lb. potatoes, MA
33.5 lb. oats in KY	35 lb. oats in MO	56 lb. potatoes, NC
50 lb. pears	22 lb. peanuts	56 lb. potatoes, VA
60 lb. dried peas	56 lb. green peas	

Which is heavier, an ounce of gold or an ounce of feathers?
What is heavier, a pound of gold or a pound of feathers?

Gold is measured in troy ounces, where 480 grains = 1 ounce. Feathers are measured in avoirdupois, where 436.5 grains = 1 ounce. Therefore, *an ounce of gold is heavier*! In troy weight, 12 oz. = 1 pound = 5760 grains. In avoirdupois, 16 oz. = 1 pound = 6989 grains. Therefore, a *pound of feathers is heavier*!

By 1640, it was obvious to people of the world that they would have to standardize the system of measurement. A good system of measurement should be based on some unchanging, long-enduring, absolute standard that exists in the physical world. Gabriel Mouton proposed that a unit of length be based on a portion of the earth's circumference. Remember that in 1640, everyone believed the earth to be perfectly round and never-changing in size and shape. (We know now that the earth is more pear-shaped and is constantly changing shape because of tides and gravitational attraction by other planets and solar systems.) In 1641, Jean Picard suggested using a pendulum. By then, the laws of physics were well established. He suggested that the length of a pendulum that takes exactly 1 second to make a complete swing be used as the standard unit of length. The metric system, developed in 1790, used Mouton's idea, and the *meter* was defined as one forty-millionth of the earth's circumference. Because Mouton was the first to suggest using the earth's circumference, he is considered the "father of the metric system."

A Brief History of the Metric System

In 1790, a group of scientists at the French Academy of Science (the best in the world at that time) proposed a complete system of measurement based on Mouton's idea. They took one forty-millionth of the earth's circumference and named it a *meter*. They related a unit of volume to length—the cubic metre was called a *stere*. Square land measurement (10 m × 10 m) was called an *are*. They took a right angle and divided it into 100 degrees (instead of 90°) and called it a *grade* (the word centigrade referred to angle degrees). They even proposed changing the calendar to a ten-day week (instead of seven). In French history, France operated under a ten-day week calendar from 1836–1838. The metric measurement system did not become popular until the ten-day week calendar was dropped. In 1840, France officially adopted the metric system as its only system of measurement.

In 1790, the United States, then a new country, was led by President George Washington and Secretary of State Thomas Jefferson. At the First Continental Congress, Jefferson introduced two bills into Congress. The first proposed adopting a decimal system of coinage—dollars, dimes, cents, mills, and 10, 100, and 1000 multiples of a dollar. This bill passed. The second bill proposed adopting a decimal system of measurement, keeping a foot, but dividing it into 10ths instead of 12ths, and dividing inches into 10ths, or adopting the newly proposed French metric system. The bill failed, and, as a result, the United States inherited the cumbersome English system of measurement.

Since 1840, one country after another has adopted the metric system, and now the U.S. is the only major industrial nation still handicapped with the outdated and inefficient English system. However, in 1957, the U.S. Armed Forces, and in 1959, the pharmaceutical association, switched to the metric system. Our two biggest exports, autos and computers, are now totally metric.

In 1960, the Eleventh International Conference on Weights and Measures made some significant changes in the metric system. The changes included: renaming the metric system *Le Système International d'Unités* or **SI**; adopting the "re" spelling (as in litre and metre), redefining the meter as 1,650,763.73 wavelengths of Krypton 86 in vacuo (defining the meter atomically rather than as a portion of the earth's circumference); increasing the list of prefixes so that more accurate scientific measurements would have meaning; and adopting time in seconds as the seventh base unit.

These conferences have been taking place periodically since 1875, when the U.S. signed the *Treaty of the Metre* agreeing to go metric. The most recent conferences took place in 1980 and 1985. Among the changes made in SI at these conferences was an expanded list of prefixes. SI is an evolving, changing system of measurement. This flexibility is the key to its worldwide success.

```
┌──────────────────────────────────────────────────┐
│                  BASE UNITS IN SI                  │
├──────────────────────────────────────────────────┤
│                  length = meter (m)                │
│          mass (weight) = kilogram (kg)             │
│                    time = second (s)               │
│       temperature = degrees Celsius (°C)           │
│      amount of substance = mole (mol)              │
│        electrical current = ampere (A)             │
│       luminous intensity = candella (cd)           │
│    volume (a related unit) = liter (l = L)         │
└──────────────────────────────────────────────────┘
```

Metric Prefixes

Multiple in decimal form	Power of 10	Prefix	Symbol	Pronunciation	Meaning
1 000 000 000 000 000	10^{15}	exa	A	ĕx′ ă	one quatrillion times base
1 000 000 000 000	10^{12}	tera	T	tĕr′ ă	one trillion times base
1 000 000 000	10^{9}	giga	G	jĭg′ ă	one billion times base
10 000 000	10^{7}	myria	my	mī′ rē ah	ten million times base
1 000 000	10^{6}	mega	M	mĕg′ ă	one million times base
1 000	10^{3}	kilo	k	kĭl′ ō	one thousand times base
100	10^{2}	hecto	h	hĕk′ tō	one hundred times base
10	10^{1}	deka	da	dĕk′ ă	ten times base
1	10^{0}	**base unit**			
0.1	10^{-1}	deci	d	dĕs′ ĭ	one tenth times base
0.01	10^{-2}	centi	c	sĕnt′ ĭ	one hundredth times base
0.001	10^{-3}	milli	m	mĭl′ ĭ	one thousandth times base
0.000001	10^{-6}	micro	μ	mī′ krō	one millionth times base
0.000000001	10^{-9}	nano	n	năn′ ō	one billionth times base
0.000000000001	10^{-12}	pico	p	pē′ kō	one trillionth times base
0.000000000000001	10^{-15}	femto	f	fĕm′ tō	one quatrillionth times base
.000000000000000001	10^{-18}	atto	a	ă′ tō	one quintillionth times base

Appendix B

Tables

Table 1. Internal Conversions

Apothecaries' Weights	Apothecaries' Measures	Household Measures	Metric Measures
60 grains = 1 dram 8 drams = 1 ounce	60 minims = 1 dram 8 drams = 1 ounce 16 oz. = 1 pint 32 oz. = 1 quart 2 pints = 1 quart 4 quarts = 1 gallon	3 tsp. = 1 Tbl. 2 Tbl. = 1 oz 8 oz. = 1 cup 2 cups = 1 pint	(for metric conversion use chart) *or:* 1000 μg = 1 mg 1000 mg = 1 g 1000 g = 1 kg 100 cm = 1 m

Table 2. Metric Conversions Using Prefixes

Metric Conversion Chart
kilo-, hecto-, deka-   meter liter   deci-, centi-, milli- gram
Move the decimal point the same number of places and in the same direction the unit moves on the chart.

Table 3. Approximate Equivalents

Apothecaries' System		Metric System
15 or 16 minims	=	1 ml, cc
1 fluid dram (f ℨ)	=	4 ml
1 dram	=	4 grams
1 fluid ounce (f ℥)	=	30 ml
1 ounce	=	30 grams
1 pint	=	500 ml
1 quart	=	1000 ml = 1 liter
15 or 16 grains	=	1 gram
1 grain	=	60–65 mg
2.2 pounds	=	1 kg
Household	Apothecaries'	Metric
1 tsp. = 5 ml	1 dram	= 4 ml
1 Tbl. = 3 tsp.	= 4 drams	= 15 or 16 ml
2 Tbl. = 8 drams	= 1 ounce	= 30 ml

Table 4. Approximate Equivalents (precise to three decimal places)

Apothecaries' System		Metric System
16.231 minims	=	1 ml, cc
1 fluid dram	=	3.697 ml
1 dram	=	3.888 grams
1 fluid ounce	=	29.574 ml
1 ounce	=	31.103 grams
1 pint	=	473.163 ml
1 quart	=	0.946 liter = 946 ml
15.432 grains	=	1 gram
1 grain	=	64.799 mg
2.205 pounds	=	1 kilogram

NOMOGRAM
(Courtesy Abbott Laboratories)

HEIGHT		SURFACE AREA	WEIGHT ·	
feet	centimeters	in square meters	pounds	kilograms

HEIGHT — feet / centimeters:

7' — 220, 215
10" — 210
8" — 205
6" — 200
4" — 195
2" — 190
6' — 185
10" — 180, 175
8" — 170
6" — 165
4" — 160
2" — 155
5' — 150
10" — 145
8" — 140
6" — 135
4" — 130
2" — 125
4' — 120
10" — 115
8" — 110
6" — 105
4" — 100
2" — 95
3' — 90
10" — 85
8" — 80
6" — 75

SURFACE AREA — in square meters:

3.00, 2.90, 2.80, 2.70, 2.60, 2.50, 2.40, 2.30, 2.20, 2.10, 2.00, 1.95, 1.90, 1.85, 1.80, 1.75, 1.70, 1.65, 1.60, 1.55, 1.50, 1.45, 1.40, 1.35, 1.30, 1.25, 1.20, 1.15, 1.10, 1.05, 1.00, .95, .90, .85, .80, .75, .70, .65, .60

WEIGHT — pounds / kilograms:

440 — 200
420 — 190
400 — 180
380 — 170
360 — 160
340 — 150
320 — 140
300
290 — 130
280
270 — 120
260
250
240 — 110
230
220 — 100
210 — 95
200 — 90
190 — 85
180 — 80
170
160 — 75
150 — 70
140 — 65
130 — 60
120 — 55
110 — 50
100 — 45
90 — 40
80 — 35
70 — 30
60 — 25
50 — 20

Appendix C

Pediatric Formulas

During the past ten years, pharmaceutical companies have responded to pediatricians' requests to produce medications with pediatric dosages in terms of body weight. Today, Fried's, Young's, and Clark's rules for figuring pediatric dosages are rarely used. The nomogram is still used by cardiologists, hematologists, oncologists, and endocrinologists for situations in which drug therapy would require a more precise dosage calculation by body surface area. Fried's, Young's, Clark's, and body surface area rules are presented here for your reference.

Fried's rule. (for infants younger than 1 year)

This formula gives a fractional part of the adult dosages. Think of 150 in the formula as months. If 150 is divided by 12 months (1 year), we get $12\frac{1}{2}$ years, the age at which most children are given adult dosages.

$$\textbf{Infant Dosage} = \frac{\textbf{age in months}}{\textbf{150}} \times \textbf{Adult Dosage}$$

Young's rule. (for children greater than 1 year, but less than 12 years old)

Adding 12 to the child's age in the denominator of the formula below yields a fractional part of the adult dosage.

$$\textbf{Child Dosage} = \frac{\textbf{age in years}}{\textbf{age of child} + \textbf{12}} \times \textbf{Adult Dosage}$$

Clark's rule. (for children greater than 1 year, but less than 12 years old)

Notice that 150 in the first formula and 70 in the second formula would represent average adult weight in pounds and kilograms, respectively. These formulas also find a fractional part of the adult dosage.

$$\text{Child Dosage} = \frac{\text{weight in pounds}}{150} \times \text{Adult Dosage}$$

$$\text{Child Dosage} = \frac{\text{weight in kilograms}}{70} \times \text{Adult Dosage}$$

Body surface area rule. (for children greater than 1 year old)
The numerator in this formula is the child's body surface area obtained from the nomogram. The 1.73 in the denominator represents the body surface area of an average adult. This formula also finds a fractional part of the adult dose, and is considered more accurate since it uses both the child's height and weight.

$$\text{Child Dosage} = \frac{\text{child's surface area in m}^2}{1.73} \times \text{Adult Dosage}$$

Appendix D

Cumulative Review

Answers to these problems are found in the Answer section at the end of the book.

Chapters 1, 2, 3—Arithmetic Operations

1. $3\frac{1}{4} + 2\frac{3}{8} + 1\frac{1}{2} =$ _____

2. $12\frac{1}{4} - 9\frac{3}{4} =$ _____

3. $\frac{1}{4} \times 2\frac{1}{2} =$ _____

4. $\frac{14}{15} \div 2\frac{1}{3} =$ _____

5. $0.0894 \div 0.03 =$ _____

6. $6.04 \times 0.15 =$ _____

7. $0.04 + 2.6 + 3 + 1.058 =$ _____

8. Change $\frac{26}{4}$ to a mixed number. _____

9. Change $5\frac{3}{8}$ to an improper fraction. _____

10. Change 0.2 to a percent. _____

11. Change 45% to a reduced fraction. _____

12. Change $\frac{3}{8}$ to a decimal. _____

13. Round 83.45928 to the nearest unit (one). _____

14. Round 83.45928 to the nearest tenth. _____

15. Round 83.45928 to the nearest hundredth. _____

16. Round 83.45928 to the nearest thousandth. _____

17. Reduce $\dfrac{\frac{1}{4}}{\frac{3}{8}}$ _____

18. Change $\frac{1}{250}$ to a percent. _____

19. Change $2\frac{1}{2}\%$ to a decimal. _____

Solve these proportions:

20. $\dfrac{3}{8} = \dfrac{X}{48}$ 21. $\dfrac{X}{5} = \dfrac{3.20}{4.5}$ 22. $\dfrac{\frac{1}{4}}{\frac{1}{2}} = \dfrac{8}{X}$

23. The doctor orders 5 grains of a drug per day. The drug comes in tablets containing $1\frac{1}{4}$ grains each. How many tablets should the patient receive per day?

24.   You give a patient $\frac{1}{3}$ oz. q.4h. How many ounces does he get in one day?

25.   You give a patient $1\frac{1}{2}$ tablets from a bottle labeled 350 mg each. How many mg did he receive?

26.   A label reads: "Give 2 mg for every 5 kg of body weight." If the patient weighs 48 kg, how many mg should you give?

27.   The doctor has ordered 5 mg VALIUM® (diazepam) t.i.d. The tablets on hand are of 2.5 mg strength. How many tablets has the patient received at the end of the day?

_____

Space Provided for Student Work

_____

Chapters 4, 5, 6—Systems of Measurement

Chart these dosages using the appropriate symbols or abbreviations and the appropriate numerals (Roman and Arabic).

28.   One and one-half drams   _____

29.   One and one-half liters   _____

30.   One-fourth ounce   _____

31.   ten minims   _____

32.   fifteen grains   _____

33.   fifteen grams   _____

34.   two and one-half milligrams   _____

35.   two teaspoons   _____

36.   two tablets   _____

37.   thirty-five kilograms   _____

38.   Given the following formulas:

$$°F = \frac{9}{5}°C = 32 \qquad °C = \frac{5}{9}(°F - 32)$$

Use the correct formula to convert a patient's temp of 40.5°C to °F.

Complete the following conversions. Use one of the conversion methods discussed in the text.

39.   30 ℳ = _____ ml   40.   2500 ml = _____ qt.

41. $2\frac{1}{2}$ oz. = _____ dr.   42.   0.45 g = _____ mg

43.   45 gr. = _____ dr.   44.   160 oz. = _____ qt.

45.   350 g = _____ kg   46. $1\frac{1}{2}$ tsp. = _____ cc

47.   16 dr. = _____ Tbls.   48.   8 gr. = _____ g

49.   125 mg = _____ gr.   50. $\frac{1}{2}$ dr. = _____ ℳ$_x$

Solve the following problems.

51.   Ordered: gr. $\frac{1}{5}$ q.d. to be given in divided doses t.i.d.
      Available: tablets, 2 mg each
      Give _____ tablets.

52.   Ordered   400 mg q.a.m.
      Available: tablets, 0.2 g each
      Give _____ tablets

53.   Ordered: gr. viii q.p.m.
      Available: tablets, 0.5 g each
      Give _____ tablets.

54.   An infant consumes 4 oz. of formula per feeding. The formula is supplied in 180 ml cans. If the infant is fed q.4h., how many cans are needed for three days?

55.   If 3 ml of blood contains 2.5 g of hemoglobin, how many grams of hemoglobin would you expect to find in 2 ml of blood?

56.   A ten-year old child weighs 64 pounds. You are to give 5 mg of Amino-phylline for every kg of body weight. How many milligrams should you give?

Chapter 7, 8   Dosages, Solutions and IV rates

57.   Ordered: sodium heparin 4000 U SQ
Available: 5 ml vial labeled 10 000 U/ml
Patient dosage: _____

58.   Ordered: procaine hydrochloride 500 mg
Label: procaine hydrochloride: 15% solution
Patient dosage: _____

59.   Ordered: erythromycin 125 mg P.O. q.6h.
Label:

```
┌──────────────────────────────────┐
│            100 ml vial           │
│       ILOSONE LIQUID®            │
│       erythromycin estolate      │
│       oral suspension, USP       │
│          250 mg per 5 ml         │
└──────────────────────────────────┘
```

Patient dosage: _____

60.   Ordered: DEMEROL® (meperidine hydrochloride) 75 mg
Available: vial labeled 50 mg/ml
Patient dosage: _____

61.   Ordered: epinephrine   10 μg per kg body mass
Patient weight: 77 pounds
Available: 1 : 1000 solution
Patient dosage: _____

62. Ordered: VISTARIL® 50 mg P.O. q.i.d.
     Label:

> 120 ml vial
> VISTARIL®
> hydroxyzine pamoate
> oral suspension
> 25 mg/5 ml

Patient dosage: _____

63. Ordered: morphine sulfate gr. $\frac{1}{4}$
     Label:

> 20 dosette vials–each contains 1 ml
> MORPHINE
> SULFATE INJECTION, USP
> 15 mg/ml

Patient dosage: _____

64. Ordered: 60 U of U-100 insulin
     Calculate how much to give from a syringe marked in cc's. _____

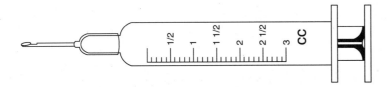

65. Ordered: MONOCID® 500 mg IM b.i.d.
     Label:

> 500 mg vial
> MONOCID®
> (sterile cefonicid sodium [lyophilized])
> Use 2.0 ml diluent   total volume 2.2 ml
> 225 mg/ml

Patient·dosage: _____
What should you do with this vial? _____

66. Ordered: TAZICEF® 30 mg/kg body mass IV q.8h.
    Child's weight: 22 pounds
    Label:

    ```
    6 gram bulk vial
    TAZICEF®
    (ceftazidime) for injection
    26 ml diluent        volume 30 ml
    ```

    Patient dosage: _____

    What should you do with this vial? _____

67. Ordered: ANCEF® 250 mg IM q.i.d.
    Label:

    ```
    5 gram bulk vial
    ANCEF®
    (sterile cefazolin sodium [lyophilized])
    Diluent 23 ml       Volume 26 ml
    1 g/5 ml
    ```

    Patient dosage: _____

    What should you do with this vial? _____

68. Ordered: potassium penicillin G 150 000 U IM
    Available: vial of powdered potassium penicillin G: 1 000 000 U
       add 9.6 ml diluent to provide 100 000 U/ml
       add 4.6 ml diluent to provide 200 000 U/ml
       add 3.6 ml diluent to provide 250 000 U/ml

    Which strength will you administer? _____

    Patient dosage: _____

69. How many grams of sodium chloride are contained in 500 ml of 0.9% saline
    solution?

70. Concentrated sodium chloride solution has a strength of 23.4%. How many ml would you add to sterile water to prepare 300 ml of normal saline solution (0.9% strength).

71. ZEPHIRAN® Chloride (benzalkoniun chloride) Antiseptic is available in a 17% concentration. How many ml of this concentrate are needed to prepare 400 ml of 0.1% solution?

72. Ordered: IV 0.45% saline 1000 ml q.8h.
    Drop factor: 15 gtts./ml
    IV rate of flow: _____

73. Ordered: IV 5% D/W at 120 ml/hr.
    Drop factor: 20 gtts./ml
    IV rate of flow: _____

74. Ordered: IV medication diluted to 50 ml. Infuse over 40 minutes and follow with a 15 ml flush.
    Label: 30 mg/ml
    Pediatric drop factor: 60 gtts./ml
    IV rate of flow: _____

75. Ordered: IV 1000 ml 10% D/W
    Drop factor: 15 gtts./ml
    Rate of flow: 45 gtts./min.
    How long will this IV run?   _____

76. Ordered: 2000 ml IV fluids in 16 hours plus piggyback medication in 100 ml to run 60 min. q.8h.
    Drop factor: 20 gtts./ml
    What is the rate of flow for each piggyback?   _____

    What is the rate of flow for the IV between piggybacks?   _____

77.   Ordered: IV medication diluted to 10 ml. Infuse over 10 minutes
                        and follow with a 15 ml flush.
      Label: 5 mg/2 ml
      Pediatric drop factor: 60 gtts./ml
      IV rate of flow: _____

78.   Ordered: AMOXIL® t.i.d.
      Child's weight: 35 pounds
      Label: AMOXIL® 20 mg/kg/day
      How many mg should you give this child per dose?   _____

79.   Ordered: ILOSONE® q.i.d.
      Child's weight: 45 pounds
      Label: ILOSONE® (erythromycin estolate) 50 mg/kg/day
      How many mg should you give this child per dose?   _____

80.   Ordered: ANCEF® q.i.d.
      Child's weight: 32 kg
      Label: ANCEF®(sterile cefazoline sodium [lyophilized]) 100 mg/kg/day
      How many mg should you give this child per dose?   _____

81.   Ordered: ADRIAMYCIN RDF® as a one-time dose
      Patient's height and weight: 52 in.; 85 lb.
      Label: ADRIAMYCIN RDF®(doxorubicin hydrochloride) 20 mg/m^2
      How many mg should the patient be given?   _____

82.   Ordered: LIDOCAINE® 2 g IV in 250 ml 5% D/W to run at 2 mg/min.
      Find the drug infusion rate in ml/min. and ml/hr.

83.   Ordered: DOPAMINE® 400 mg IV in 250 ml 5% D/W to run at 40 mg/hr.
      Find the drug infusion rate in ml/min. and ml/hr.

Answers

Chapter 1

1.1 (pp. 4–5)

1) $\frac{1}{6}$ 2) $\frac{8}{6}$ 3) $\frac{3}{6}$ 4) $\frac{5}{4}$ 5) proper   6) improper

7) proper   8) mixed   9) mixed   10) improper   11) improper

12) proper   13) $\frac{4}{16}$ 14) $\frac{8}{12}$

1.2 (pp. 9–11)

1) $6\frac{1}{2}$ 2) $2\frac{2}{7}$ 3) $4\frac{1}{4}$ 4) $11\frac{2}{3}$ 5) $7\frac{5}{9}$ 6) $2\frac{7}{16}$ 7) $2\frac{5}{8}$

8) $1\frac{6}{17}$ 9) $\frac{27}{4}$ 10) $\frac{86}{17}$ 11) $\frac{80}{11}$ 12) $\frac{17}{3}$ 13) $\frac{56}{9}$ 14) $\frac{9}{1}$

15) $\frac{58}{5}$ 16) $\frac{87}{4}$ 17) 10   18) 15   19) 28   20) 24   21) 9

22) 48   23) $\frac{3}{5}$ 24) $\frac{1}{9}$ 25) $\frac{2}{3}$ 26) $\frac{3}{4}$ 27) $\frac{7}{6}$ or $1\frac{1}{6}$ 28) $\frac{7}{10}$

29) $\frac{2}{5}$ 30) $\frac{5}{7}$ 31) $5\frac{1}{4}$ 32) $2\frac{1}{8}$ 33) 7   34) $4\frac{1}{6}$ 35) $4\frac{1}{2}$

36) $9\frac{2}{5}$ 37) 15   38) $4\frac{1}{2}$

1.3 (pp. 16–17)

1) $1\frac{7}{12}$ 2) $1\frac{1}{12}$ 3) $1\frac{7}{40}$ 4) $1\frac{23}{24}$ 5) $1\frac{17}{24}$ 6) $\frac{29}{30}$ 7) $1\frac{1}{12}$

8) $9\frac{2}{3}$ 9) $15\frac{5}{8}$ 10) $18\frac{7}{12}$ 11) $7\frac{14}{15}$ 12) $4\frac{13}{24}$ 13) $6\frac{7}{12}$

14) $9\frac{9}{10}$ 15) $11\frac{19}{24}$ 16) $\frac{3}{20}$ 17) $\frac{1}{8}$ 18) $\frac{1}{12}$ 19) $\frac{4}{15}$ 20) $\frac{11}{18}$

21) $\frac{4}{21}$ 22) $11\frac{3}{5}$ 23) $2\frac{1}{14}$ 24) $3\frac{1}{8}$ 25) $1\frac{19}{24}$ 26) $4\frac{1}{2}$

27) $4\frac{23}{24}$ 28) $1\frac{3}{4}$ miles   29) $13\frac{1}{2}$ pounds

1.4 (pp. 21–22)

1) $\frac{2}{9}$ 2) $\frac{3}{8}$ 3) $\frac{4}{35}$ 4) 2   5) $2\frac{2}{3}$ 6) $1\frac{5}{7}$ 7) $\frac{2}{7}$ 8) $1\frac{2}{5}$

9) $\frac{1}{2}$ 10) $1\frac{9}{16}$ 11) $1\frac{1}{3}$ 12) 2   13) 20   14) $\frac{5}{6}$ 15) 2

16) $\frac{2}{27}$ 17) 15   18) 12   19) $2\frac{4}{5}$ 20) $\frac{1}{81}$ 21) $\frac{9}{14}$ 22) 4

23) 1   24) $1\frac{3}{7}$ 25) $10\frac{1}{2}$ tablets   26) 5 days

1.5 (pp. 23–26)

1) $\frac{1}{5}$ taken   2) $\frac{2}{3}$ left   3) 9 packets   4) 6 oz.   5) $\frac{1}{8}$ gr.   6) $\frac{1}{2}$ tab.

7) $\frac{1}{4}$ tab.   8) 12 gr.   9) 45 mg   10) $1\frac{1}{2}$ tab.   11) $2\frac{1}{2}$ gr.   12) 5 gr.

13) 2 tab.   14) $2\frac{1}{2}$ tab.   15) $\frac{17}{18}$ 16) $1\frac{1}{2}$ mile   17) $160\frac{5}{8}$ lbs.

18) 134 lbs.   19) $6\frac{7}{8}$ gr.   20) 18 oz.   21) $1\frac{3}{4}$ oz.   22) 8 oz.

23) 3 gr.   24) $2\frac{11}{12}$ mi.

Chapter 1 Test (pp. 27–28)

1) $1\frac{13}{40}$ 2) $7\frac{14}{15}$ 3) $\frac{3}{8}$ 4) $5\frac{3}{7}$ 5) $2\frac{5}{8}$ 6) $1\frac{1}{3}$ 7) 24

8) $\frac{1}{3}$ 9) 2   10) 4 tab.   11) 2 cc   12) $12\frac{7}{8}$ gr.   13) $1\frac{1}{2}$ gr.

14) 50 mg   15) 27 mg   16) 25 mg   17) $7\frac{1}{2}$ ml   18) 4 tab.

19) 4 tab.   20) $1\frac{1}{2}$ tab.

Chapter 2

2.1 (pp. 32–34)

1) three hundredths   2) two hundred fifty-seven thousandths
3) three and four thousandths   4) twenty-six and two tenths
5) one hundred twenty-five and three hundred seventy-five thousandths
6) thirty-five ten-thousandths   7) six and twenty-five hundredths
8) eight ten-thousandths   9) 6.034   10) 0.051   11) 0.0165
12) 120   13) 45.6   14) 900.09   15) 0.89   16) 30.5   17) 0.3
18) 2.4   19) 34.6   20) 0.3   21) 125.37   22) 0.04   23) 23.67
24) 0.01   25) 56.785   26) 0.007   27) 0.765   28) 78.084
29) 6774.4   30) 6800   31) 6774.353   32) 6774.35   33) 6774
34) 7000   35) 6770   36) 6774.3528

2.2 (pp. 36–38)

1) 1.4   2) 7.851   3) 0.46   4) 25.34   5) 6.01   6) 1.21
7) 24.834   8) 30.965   9) 13.02   10) 4.444   11) 1918.49

12) 411.166   13) 7.3   14) 0.2   15) 1.85   16) 33.99   17) 2.063
18) 11.1   19) 20   20) 16.4975   21) 2.98   22) 154.14
23) 85.18   24) 302.45   25) 1.11   26) 11.4   27) 7.63   28) 32.7
29) 5.35 mile   30) 13.5 lbs.   31) 0.41 kg   32) 14.45 oz.

2.3 (pp. 42–44)

1) 0.12006   2) 0.20024   3) 0.00014   4) 5.125   5) 0.008
6) 25.6   7) 5.32   8) 1.95   9) 0.06   10) 1.5625   11) 6.25
12) 28.875   13) 8.15   14) 0.08   15) 0.125   16) 2.15   17) 7
18) 10470   19) 245   20) 2.15   21) 0.33   22) 0.04   23) 35.59
24) 3.56   25) 0.2848   26) 0.256   27) 1.9   28) 0.4   29) 45 gr.
30) 4 days   31) 11 doses   32) 3 mg

2.4 (pp. 49–50)

1) 0.2   2) 0.875   3) 0.025   4) 0.12   5) 0.67   6) 0.43
7) 3.375   8) 4.33   9) 8.75   10) 2.3125   11) 1.3   12) 3.375
13) 21.25   14) 3.75   15) 0.08   16) 5.83   17) 1.6   18) 0.017
19) 3.25   20) 0.001   21) $\frac{4}{5}$ 22) $\frac{13}{20}$ 23) $\frac{33}{100}$ 24) $\frac{3}{500}$
25) $\frac{3}{250}$ 26) $4\frac{2}{5}$ 27) $2\frac{1}{2}$ 28) $2\frac{1}{20}$ 29) $\frac{3}{8}$ 30) $1\frac{1}{250}$
31) $\frac{8}{1}$ 32) $12\frac{3}{10}$ 33) $\frac{9}{25}$ 34) $20\frac{3}{2500}$ 35) $\frac{1}{40}$ 36) $\frac{1}{800}$
37) 1.75, $1\frac{3}{4}$ 38) 1.875, $1\frac{7}{8}$ 39) $8\frac{1}{5}$, 8.2   40) 1.125, $1\frac{1}{8}$

2.5 (pp. 53–55)

1) 33%   2) 65%   3) 28%   4) 86%   5) 25%   6) 12.5%
7) 37.5%   8) 12.75%   9) 0.75%   10) 4.85%   11) 30%   12) 40%
13) 80%   14) 110%   15) 150%   16) 5%   17) 3%   18) 280%
19) 50%   20) 2%   21) 0.27   22) 0.85   23) 0.17   24) 0.05
25) 0.16   26) 0.03   27) 0.065   28) 0.0165   29) 0.1285   30) 0.003
31) 1.3   32) 2.5   33) 0.6   34) 0.092   35) 0.0005   36) 0.0001
37) 0.0025   38) 0.021   39) 0.008   40) 0.089   41) 0.00125
42) 0.125   43) 0.0125   44) 0.072   45) $0.00\overline{6}$ or 0.0067
46) 0.375   47) 0.04375   48) 0.0283   49) 0.0075   50) 0.066

2.6 (pp. 60–62)

1) 2.5%   2) 73.3%   3) 240%   4) 80%   5) 2%   6) 112.5%
7) 28.6%   8) 37.5%   9) 15%   10) 0.25%   11) 25%   12) 18.75%
13) 66.7%   14) 5%   15) 0.1%   16) $\frac{1}{4}$ 17) 3   18) $\frac{3}{20}$ 19) $\frac{1}{5}$
20) $\frac{2}{25}$ 21) $\frac{4}{5}$ 22) $\frac{1}{200}$ 23) $\frac{1}{20000}$ 24) $\frac{1}{2000}$ 25) $\frac{1}{40}$
26) $\frac{3}{800}$ 27) $\frac{3}{8}$ 28) $\frac{1}{16}$ 29) $\frac{1}{3}$ 30) $\frac{1}{200}$ 31) $\frac{3}{40}$ 32) $\frac{1}{16}$
33) $\frac{1}{25}$ 34) $1\frac{1}{2}$ 35) $\frac{1}{500}$

36) [table]

$\frac{3}{40}$	0.075	7.5%		$\frac{1}{40}$	**0.025**	2.5%
$\frac{9}{20}$	**0.45**	45%		$\frac{1}{20}$	0.05	5%
$\frac{3}{400}$	0.0075	$\frac{3}{4}$%		$\frac{1}{4}$	0.25	**25%**
$2\frac{1}{5}$	2.2	220%		$3\frac{1}{5}$	**3.2**	320%
$\frac{1}{125}$	**0.008**	0.8%		$\frac{3}{1000}$	0.003	**0.3%**

37) $66\frac{2}{3}$% or 66.7%   38) 20%   39) 25%   40) 3.3%

2.7 (pp. 65–67)

1) 3.125 mg   2) 116.25 mg   3) 0.625% or $\frac{5}{8}$%   4) 25%   5) 3 mg
6) 1.8 mg   7) 6.5 ml   8) 7.5 hr.   9) 170.25 lbs., 9.25 lbs.   10) 12.5 mg
11) 2.5 mg   12) 2.5 mg   13) 20.3 miles   14) 29.7 miles
15) 2.5 oz.   16) 41.25 hr.   17) 1.25 hr.   18) 7.5 hr.   9) 8 lbs.
20) 350 mg   21) 42 mg   22) 2.5 mg   23) 3.75 lbs.   24) 25%
25) 0.5%   26) 199 lbs. 6 oz. or 199.375 lbs., 26 lbs. 6 oz. or 26.375 lbs.
27) 2 tab.

Chapter 2 Test (pp. 68–70)

1) 1255.6   2) 1300   3) 1255.625   4) 1255.63   5) 60.175
6) 7.25   7) 0.48   8) 0.33   9) 3.34   10) 0.04   11) 0.1875
12) 3.93   13) 16.672   14) 26.875   15) 3.045   16) 3.303
17) 2.6, $2\frac{3}{5}$ 18) 0.375, $\frac{3}{8}$ 19) 0.75, $\frac{3}{4}$

20) [table]

$\frac{7}{40}$	0.175	17.5%		$\frac{1}{2000}$	**0.0005**	0.05%
$\frac{17}{20}$	**0.85**	85%		$\frac{7}{500}$	0.014	1.4%
$1\frac{1}{5}$	1.2	120%		$\frac{1}{10000}$	0.0001	**0.01%**
$\frac{3}{100}$	0.03	**3%**		$\frac{2}{125}$	0.016	$1\frac{3}{5}$%

21) 10.05 mi.   22) under, 1.95 mi.   23) 6 lbs. 7.1 oz   24) 18.75 mg
25) 0.45 mg   26) 2.5 mg   27) 3 tab.   28) 18 doses, no   29) 7 days
30) 2.5%

Chapter 3

3.1 (pp. 74–77)

1) $\frac{1}{8}$ 2) $\frac{2}{13}$ 3) $\frac{1}{9}$ 4) $\frac{2}{7}$ 5) $\frac{9}{2}$ 6) $\frac{3}{4}$ 7) $\frac{3}{4}$ 8) $\frac{9}{2}$ 9 $\frac{5}{8}$

10) $\frac{1}{20}$ 11) 45:26   12) 3:4000   13) 8:5   14) 1:3   15) 3:10

16) 4 to 3   17) 1 to 4   18) 8 to 9   19) 6 ft./min.   20) $\frac{1\ \text{women}}{5\ \text{men}}$

21) 83.3 ml/hr. or $\frac{250\ \text{ml}}{3\ \text{hr.}}$ 22) 3 ml:200 mg or 0.015 ml/mg

23) 100 ml/hr.   24) 3 women to 4 men   25) 0.5 mg/ml

26) 1.5 mg/ml   27) 41.7 ml/hr.   28) 125 ml/hr.

29) 12.5 mg/ml   30) 5 men to 17 patients

3.2 (pp. 80–82)

1) no   2) no   3) yes   4) no   5) yes   6) no   7) yes   8) no

9) yes   10) yes   11) 2.5 or $2\frac{1}{2}$ 12) 30   13) 126   14) 2

15) 2   16) 1.6   17) $5\frac{1}{3}$ 18) $\frac{2}{7}$ 19) 8   20) 16   21) $7\frac{1}{2}$

22) 4   23) $1\frac{2}{3}$ 24) 2.5   25) 0.2   26) $83\frac{1}{3}$ or $83.\overline{3}$ 27) 0.3

28) 4   29) 3   30) 50

3.3 (pp. 86–88)

1) 8 grams to 100 ml   2) 24 grams/100 ml   3) $7\frac{1}{2}$ grams in 100 ml

4) 8 grams = 50 ml   5) 1 g to 100 ml   6) $\frac{15\ \text{g}}{200\ \text{ml}}$ 7) 2.5%

8) 75%   9) 6.7% or $6\frac{2}{3}$%   10) 0.01%   11) 0.4%   12) 1%

13) 2%   14) 0.025%   15) 2%   16) 0.07%   17) 0.05%   18) 0.2%

19) $\frac{1}{10}$ 20) $\frac{3}{40}$ 21) $\frac{21}{400}$ 22) 3:200   23) 1:400   24) 1:100 000

25) 1:2500   26) 1 g/40 ml   27) 1 g/8 ml   28) 1:300   29) 1:200

30) 1:2000

3.4 (pp. 91–92)

1) 300 ml   2) 4 tsp.   3) 4 tab.   4) $2\frac{1}{2}$ tab.   5) 470 mg

6) 208 mg   7) 750 mg   8) 0.9 ml   9) 1.3 ml   10) 3.75 or 3.8 ml

11) 36 oz., 5 bottles   12) 18.75 g or 18.8 g

13) 1700 mg/day, 425 mg/dose   14) 1.5 ml   15) 1.5 tab.

Chapter 3 Test (pp. 93–94)

1) $\frac{16}{5}$ 2) $\frac{2}{3}$ 3) $\frac{3}{4}$ 4) 35 mg/ml   5) $\frac{5}{32}$ 6) $6\frac{2}{3}$ 7) 8.4

8) 1.22   9) 0.25   10) 0.7875   11) 0.2%   12) 6.7% or $6\frac{2}{3}$%

13) 10%   14) 6%   15) $\frac{7}{200}$ 16) 1:600   17) 1:5000   18) $\frac{21}{250}$

19) 400 ml   20) 525 mg/day, 175 mg/dose   21) 875 mg

22) 0.75 ml   23) 2.5 g   24) 5 ml   25) $\frac{1}{2}$ tab.

Chapter 4

4.3 (pp. 100–101)

1) gal.   2) oz., $\overline{3}$ or f$\overline{3}$ 3) dr., 3 or f3 4) min., ♏   5) Tbl., T
6) lbs., #   7) gtts.   8) gr.   9) qt.   10) tsp., t   11) pt.
12) c.   13) ii   14) 5   15) 8   16) x   17) xiii   18) 24
19) ix   20) ss   21) iv   22) 11   23) vi   24) xv   25) 19

4.4 (pp. 103–104)

1) 5 drams three times a day   2) 3 ounces every 4 hours

3) $6\frac{1}{2}$ minims twice a day   4) $\frac{3}{4}$ grain every morning

5) $21\frac{1}{2}$ drams every three hours   6) 2 tsp. every evening

7) $\frac{1}{2}$ pint four times a day   8) 5 grains when necessary

9) 2 quarts every day   10) 4 fluid ounces every evening
11) 2 teaspoons after meals   12) one tablet twice a day

4.5 (p. 109)

1) ss   2) $1\frac{2}{3}$ 3) iii   4) iv   5) 90   6) 480   7) 9

8) 4   9) 80   10) 60   11) $1\frac{1}{2}$ 12) 12   13) 40   14) 64

15) 48   16) $\frac{3}{4}$ 17) $2\frac{1}{2}$ 18) 16   19) 3   20) 120

4.6 (pp. 110–112)

1) 2   2) 3 3) $\frac{1}{2}$ 4) 5 qt.   5) $1\frac{1}{2}$ qt.   6) 3 qt.   7) 2 bottles

8) 4 bottles   9) $\frac{3}{4}$ oz.   10) 192 drams   11) 6 days   12) 12 oz.

13) 15 gr.   14) 15 gr.   15) 60 gr.

Chapter 4 Test (pp. 113–115)

1) ♏ viii   2) 3 v   3) $\overline{3}$ iiiss   4) f3 iss   5) gr. x   6) 2 tab.
7) 2 tsp.   8) $1\frac{1}{2}$ drams four times a day   9) 3 ounces every morning
10) 4 drams twice a day   11) 1 quart every day

12) 2 fluid drums when necessary   13) $\frac{1}{10}$ grain every day

14) $1\frac{1}{2}$ 15) $1\frac{1}{2}$ 16) 2   17) 16   18) 48   19) 16   20) $1\frac{1}{2}$

21) 48   22) 3 qt.   23) 2 oz.   24) 1 one-gallon container

25) 8 cans   26) 64 doses   27) 2 oz. left   28) 16 days   29) 5 cans

---

Chapter 5

5.1 (pp. 118–120)

1) meter   2) second   3) kilogram   4) °Celsius   5) liter

6) milli, m   7) centi, c   8) kilo, k   9) micro, μ 10) deci, d

11) 2.5 ml   12) 5 cm   13) 50 mg   14) 200 μg   15) 1.5 km

16) 300 mm   17) 2.5ml t.i.d.   18) 50mg q.h.s.   19) 0.25g q.a.m.

20) 2ℓ q.d.   21) 600μg b.i.d.   22) 52.5 cm   23) 62 kg

24) 150ml q.6h.   25) 0.5g q.4h.

26) 2.5 cubic centimeters intramuscularly three times a day

27) 30 milliliters in the morning

28) 250 micrograms per milliliter every evening

29) 5 milliliters every three hours   30) 0.375 grams when necessary

31) 500 micrograms per milliliter every hour

5.2 (pp. 125–126)

1) 9.9 cm   2) 5.1 cm   3) 14.1 cm   4) 1.1 cm   5) 7.4 cm

6) 88 cm   7) 113.5 cm   8) 0.5 cm   9) 44.5 cm   10) 19.5 cm

11) 4.5 mm   12) 6.3 cm   13) mm   14) cm   15) mm   16) cm

17) cm   18) cm   19) cm

5.3 (pp. 129–131)

1) quart   2) teaspoon   3) 2000   4) 30   5) 0.5   6) 0.25   7) 0.1

8) 250, 0.25 liter   9) 500   10) 250   11) 250   12) 2.5   13) 600

14) 3   15) 25, 25   16) 250   17) 2000   18) B   19) C   20) D

21) A   22) E   23) ml   24) ml   25) ℓ 26) ℓ 27) ml   28) ml

29) ml   30) 0.5cm^3 or 0.5cc   31) 2.5cm^2 or 2.5cc   32) 0.75ml

33) 1000ml   34) 1ℓ 35) cc   36) ml   37) ml, ℓ 38) cc

39) cc   40) ml   41) cc, ℓ 42) cc, ℓ 43) cc, ℓ

5.4 (pp. 133–134)

1) mg   2) g   3) kg   4) kg   5) g   6) mg   7) mg   8) mg

9) kg   10) g   11) 15   12) 250   13) 4   14) 2000   15) 3

16) 1500, 1500   17) 2.5   18) 72   19) 0.5   20) 500   21) 0.5

22) 1.5   23) 5.2 kg   24) 7.5g   25) 0.75g   26) 25mg   27) kg
28) μg, mg, g

5.5 (p. 136)

1) 2:30 P.M.   2) 6:00 A.M.   3) 1:00 P.M.   4) 6:15 P.M.   5) 9:30 P.M
6) 3:45 P.M.   7) 7:15 A.M.   8) 2:45 A.M.   9) 11:59 P.M. 10) 10:30 P.M.
11) 15 March 1992   12) 12 January 1989   13) 3 October 1990
14) 28 May 1991   15) 9 September 1988

5.6 (pp. 138–139)

1) G   2) E   3) D   4) C   5) A   6) F   7) B   8) 0
9) 20–22   10) 37   11) 100   12) 41   13) 39   14) 38   15) 36
16) 35   17) 38.7°C   18) 36.6°C   19) 40.4°C   20) 37.7°C

5.7 (pp. 141–142)

1) 83,000   2) 3   3) 5600   4) 0.25   5) 2000   6) 0.15
7) 0.005   8) 20,000   9) 1.65   10) 3.5   11) 180   12) 3.6
13) 0.15   14) 375   15) 0.225   16) 0.05   17) 200   18) 0.375
19) 750   20) 1.5   21) 1200   22) 675   23) 0.0035   24) 2000
25) 80   26) 4.5   27) 80 000   28) 31   29) 1.2   30) 500

5.8 (pp. 143–145)

1) 3   2) 2   3) $\frac{1}{2}$ 4) $2\frac{1}{2}$ 5) $1\frac{1}{2}$ 6) 20   7) 375 mg
8) 37.5 mg   9) 200 mg   10) 500 mg tablet
11) give 3 or 4 tablets after consulting with the doctor
12) 28 tablets   13) 5.75 g   14) 1.25 ml   15) 0.45 mg, 450 μg

Chapter 5 Test (pp. 146–147)

1) meter   2) kilogram   3) °Celsius   4) second   5) liter   6) ml
7) ℓ 8) cm^3 9) μg   10) kg   11) g   12) 0.25ml IM b.i.d.
13) 3.5cm^3 q.a.m.   14) 0.5g q.h.s.   15) 25mg q.6h.   16) 3.2 kg
17) 1000ml IV   18) 15ml p.r.n.   19) 20–22   20) 37   21) 41
22) 1   23) 5   24) 150   25) 0.075   26) 550   27) 450
28) 1.25 g   29) 5   30) 0.45   31) 0.975   32) 20 000   33) 0.02
34) 1500   35) 0715   36) 150   37) 2.5   38) 36   39) 3
40) $2\frac{1}{2}$ tablets   41) 2 tab.   42) 1.1 g   43) decimals

---

Chapter 6

6.1 (pp. 151–152)

1) 45 to 48   2) 135   3) 4 to 4.25   4) 80   5) 0.05   6) 600

7) 900 to 975   8) 5   9) 5.6 to 6   10) 3.75 to 4   11) 3

12) 68.2   13) 0.5   14) 3   15) 15   16) $\frac{1}{2}$ 17) 150   18) 120

19) 0.6 to 0.7   20) 75   21) $\frac{1}{3}$ 22) xii   23) 2.8 to 3

24) 120 to 128   25) 250   26) 1.9 to 2

6.2 (pp. 155–157)

1) 3 tab. of 100 mg strength; 2 tab. of 150 mg strength   2) 1 tab.

3) 2 capsules   4) 1   5) 2   6) 11 cans   7) 2   8) 1 ml

9) 70 kg, 350 mg   10) 2 days   11) 600 to 650 mg   12) 192–194 mg

13) $1\frac{1}{2}$ qts.   14) 8 doses   15) 3 tabs.   16) 2 tsp.   17) $\frac{1}{2}$ tsp.

18) about 6 liters   19) 557   20) 500 mg

6.3 (p. 159)

1) 41.1   2) 113   3) 57.2   4) 31.1   5) 103.1   6) 37   7) 22.2

8) 68   9) 109.4   10) 39.4   11) 0   12) 37.9

13) 35.6°F to 46.4°F

Chapter 6 Test (pp. 160–162)

1) xvi to xvii   2) 6   3) 113.6 or 120   4) 3   5) 1   6) 8   7) ℨ ī

8) f ℨ ī   9) 6 g   10) gr. 45   11) 60 kg   12) 0.4 mg   13) 4 oz.

14) 20 doses, 5 days   15) 2   16) 3   17) 2   18) 1

19) 8 kg, 40 mg   20) 9 cans   21) 900 to 975 mg   22) 3 tab.

23) 102.2   24) 39.4

Chapter 7

7.1 (pp. 164–165)

1) 2 grams of medication in every 5 ml of solution
2) 15 grams of medication in every 100 ml of solution
3) 100 units of medication in every 1 ml of solution
4) 20 mg of medication in every 1 ml of solution
5) 300 mg of medication in every 10 ml of solution
6) 1 g of medication in every 1000 ml of solution

7) 60 mg of medication in every 1 ml of solution
8) 20 g of medication in every 100 ml of solution
9) 20 mg of medication in every 3 ml of solution
10) 1 g of medication in every 10 ml of solution
11) 300 mg of medication in every 2 ml of solution
12) 50 mg of medication in every 1 ml of solution
13) 20 mEq of medication in every 15 ml of solution
14) 250 mg of medication in every 5 ml of solution
15) 25 mg of medication in every 5 ml of solution
16) 125 mg of medication in every 5 ml of solution
17) **125 mg of medication in every 5 ml of solution**

7.2 (pp. 174–178)

1) 0.5 ml	2) 0.75 ml	3) 4 ml	4) 0.6 ml	5) 4.5 ml	6) 7.5 ml
7) 0.38 ml	8) 5 ml	9) 3 ml	10) 3 ml	11) 3 ml	12) 10 ml
13) 1 ml	14) 0.2 ml	15) 0.5 ml	16) 1.5 ml	17) 1 ml	
18) 0.5 ml	19) 2.5 ml	20) 0.35 ml	21) 2 ml	22) 0.6 ml	
23) 2 ml	24) 16.7%	25) 0.08 ml	26) 0.3 ml		

7.3 (pp. 183–190)

1) 1.6 ml; every 12 hours; inject diluent to make 2 ml; discard vial
2) 1 ml; twice a day; inject diluent to make 2 ml; discard vial
3) 1 ml; every 6 hours; inject diluent to make 10 ml; relabel 100 mg = 1 ml; date, time, initials
4) 1.1 ml; every 8 hours; relabel 250 mg = 1.1 ml; date, time, initials
5) 1.5 ml; every 12 hours; inject 3.2 ml diluent; relabel 1,500,000 U = 1.5 ml; date, time, initials
6) 1 ml; every 8 hours; inject 9.6 ml diluent; relabel 100 000 U = 1 ml; date, time, initials
7) 2 ml; every 4 hours; discard vial
8) 2.5 ml; every morning; relabel 500 mg = 2.5 ml; date, time, initials
9) 2.2 ml; twice a day; use the contents of vial and discard
10) 1.5 ml; daily; relabel 500 mg = 1.5 ml; date, time, initials
11) 3 ml; daily for one week; relabel 200 mg = 3 ml; date, time, initials
12) 1.3 ml; every other day, discard vial
13) 1.25 ml; three times a day; relabel 500 mg = 1.25 ml; date, time, initials
14) 1.25 ml; every 12 hours; relabel 250 mg = 1.25 ml; date, time, initials
15) 1.5 ml; every 8 hours; relabel 300 mg = 1.5 ml; date, time, initials
16) 1.5 ml; three times a day; discard vial
17) 2.5 ml; every 8 hours; relabel 500 mg = 2.5 ml; date, time, initials
18) 1.9 ml; every 12 hours; discard vial
19) 1.4 ml; every 6 hours; relabel 385 mg = 1.4 ml; date, time, initials
20) 1.25 ml; four times a day; relabel 250 mg = 1.25 ml; date, time, initials

7.4 (pp. 192–193)

1) 3.5 g   2) 1.5 g   3) 20 g   4) 4.5 g   5) 200 mg   6) 300 mg
7) 6 ml   8) 4.5 g   9) 2 liters   10) 7.5 g   11) 25 ml

7.5 (pp. 196–198)

1) 2.9 ml of 17% solution and 497.1 ml diluent to make 500 ml total
2) 1 liter of 1:10000 solution and 1 liter diluent to make 2 liters total
3) 3.8 ml of 23.4% sodium chloride concentrate and 96.2 ml diluent to make 100 ml total
4) 9.6 ml sodium chloride concentrate and 490.4 ml diluent to make 500 ml total
5) 200 ml of 2:5 solution and 1800 ml diluent to make 2000 ml total
6) 5.9 ml of 17% solution and 994.1 ml diluent for each liter
7) 88.4 ml of 95% ethyl alcohol and 31.6 ml diluent to make 120 ml total
8) 6 ml of pure liquid cresol and 294 ml diluent to make 300 ml total
9) 2 ml of 10% solution and 18 ml diluent to make 20 ml total
10) 50 ml of pure glucose and 950 ml diluent to make 1 liter total
11) $5\frac{1}{3}$ oz. of vinegar and $122\frac{2}{3}$ oz. diluent to make 1 gal. total
12) 2:10000 or 1:5000   13) 16%   14) 0.2%   15) 0.05%
16) 9:1000
17) 125 ml of 2% mercurechrome solution and 125 ml diluent to make 250 ml total
18) 450 ml of 0.2% solution and 450 ml diluent to make 900 ml total
19) 1 ml of 5% solution and 199 ml diluent to make 200 ml total

7.6 (pp. 201–204)

1) 900 mg, 225 mg   2) 272 mg, 91 mg   3) 0.3 ml
4) 192–200 mg, 64–67 mg   5) 108 mg   6) 600 mg, 150 mg
7) 0.095 mg, 0.032 mg   8) 386 mg, 97 mg   9) 142 mg   10) 94.4 mg
11) 164 mg, 55 mg   12) 1491 mg, 373 mg   13) 227 mg
14) 1432 mg, 358 mg   15) 388 mg, 129 mg

7.7 (pp. 212–214)

1) 1.67 m^2 2) 1.85 m^2 3) 2.2 m^2 4) 0.64 m^2 5) 1.03 m^2
6) 0.87 m^2, 1.7 mg   7) 1.20 m^2, 2.4 mg   8) 1.5 m^2, 90 mg
9) 1.36 m^2, 27.2 mg   19) 1.69 m^2, 422.5 mg   11) 2.02 m^2, 505 mg
12) 0.78 m^2, 23.4 mg   13) 1.53 m^2, 92 mg

Chapter 7 Test (pp. 215–220)

1) 40 g in 100 ml   2) 1 g in 100 ml   3) 100 units per 1 ml
4) 25 mg in 2 cc or 12.5 mg/1 cc   5) 40 mEq in 30 ml
6) 15 mg in 1 ml   7) 0.4 mg per ml   8) 0.3 cc
9) 0.7 ml 4 times per day

10) 2 ml by mouth, twice a day; relabel 550 mg = 2 ml; date, time, initials

11) 0.5 cc   12) 0.45 ml   13) 4.5 ml by mouth, at bedtime

14) 7.5 ml   15) 1.5 ml to 1.7 ml

16) 1.3 ml; inject 6.8 ml diluent; relabel 80 000 U = 1.3 ml; date, time, initials

17) 1.7 oz. (51 ml) of 70% solution and 2.3 oz. (69 ml) diluent to make 4 oz. (120 ml) total

18) 14.3 ml three times a day

19) 450 ml pure glucose and 4550 ml diluent to make 5 liters total

20) 2 ml three times a day   21) 3.3 ml   22) 1.6 ml   23) $1\frac{1}{2}$ oz.

24) 0.4ml   25) 0.5 cc

26) 1.6 ml; inject 18.2 ml diluent; relabel 400 000 U = 1.6 ml; date, time, initials

27) 11.6 ml   28) 4 drops   29) 0.7 ml   30) 2 ml   31) 118 mg

32) 20 mg, 0.4 ml   33) 231 mg, 58 mg   34) 254 mg, 85 mg

35) 250 mg, 83 mg   36) 103 mg   37) 1.7 mg   38) 420 mg

Chapter 8

8.1 (pp. 225–227)

1) 31 gtts./min.   2) 50 gtts./min.   3) 25 gtts./min.

4) 12 or 13 gtts./min.   5) 33 gtts./min.   6) 67 gtts./min.

7) 42 gtts./min.   8) 37 or 38 gtts./min.   9) 100 gtts./min.

10) 50 gtts./min.   11) 31 gtts./min.   12) 42 gtts./min.

13) 62 or 63 gtts./min.   14) 28 gtts./min.   15) 62 or 63 gtts./min.

16) 83 gtts./min.   17) 125 gtts./min.   18) 33 gtts./min.

19) 21 gtts./min.   20) 31 gtts./min.

8.2 (pp. 229–231)

1) 50 gtts./min.   2) 42 gtts./min.   3) 33 gtts./min.

4) 31 gtts./min.   5) 25 gtts./min.   6) 25 gtts./min.

7) 25 gtts./min.   8) 67 gtts./min.   9) 17 gtts./min.

10) 50 gtts./min.   11) 33 gtts./min.   12) 50 gtts./min.

13) 12 or 13 gtts./min.   14) 17 gtts./min.   15) 37 or 38 gtts./min.

8.3 (p. 234)

1) 600, 10   2) 400, $6\frac{1}{2}$ 3) 484, 8   4) 1429, 24   5) 238, 4

6) 606, 10   7) 121, 2   8) 476, 8   9) 357, 6   10) 357, 6

8.4 (pp. 238–240)

1) 47 ml, 87 gtts./min.   2) 48 ml, 130 gtts./min.

3) 14 ml, 60 gtts./min.   4) 19 ml, 52 or 53 gtts./min.

5) 27 ml, 67 or 68 gtts./min.   6) 35 ml, 82 or 83 gtts./min.

7) 78 ml, 95 gtts./min.   8) 8 ml, 150 gtts./min.

9) 18 ml, 140 gtts./min.   10) 38 ml, 73 gtts./min.

8.5 (pp. 244–246)

1) 67 gtts./min., 25 gtts./min.   2) 25 gtts./min., 32 gtts./min.

3) 12 or 13 gtts./min., 35 gtts./min.   4) 33 gtts./min., 23 gtts./min.

5) 25 gtts./min., 21 gtts./min.   6) 25 gtts./min., 32 or 33 gtts./min.

7) 33 gtts./min., 27 gtts./min.   8) 25 gtts./min., 58 gtts./min.

9) 33 gts./min., 43 gtts./min.   10) 25 gtts./min., 50 gtts./min.

8.6 (pp. 250–251)

1) 1 ml/min., 60 ml/hr.   2) 2 ml/min., 120 ml/hr.

3) 0.5 ml/min., 30 ml/hr.   4) 1.17 ml/min., 70 ml/hr.

5) 12 ml/hr., 0.2 ml/min.   6) 1 ml/min., 60 ml/hr.

7) 30 ml/hr., 0.5 ml/min.   8) 0.5 ml/min., 30 ml/hr.

9) 0.75 ml/min., 45 ml/hr.   10) 80 ml/hr., 1.33 ml/min.

Chapter 8 Test (pp. 254–259)

1) 31 gtts./min.   2) 50 gtts./min.   3) 25 gtts./min.

4) 28 gtts./min.   5) 21 gtts./min.   6) 31 gtts./min.

7) 21 gtts./min.   8) 28 ml, 90 gtts./min.   9) 26 ml, 100 gtts./min.

10) 15 ml, 120 gtts./min.   11) 44 ml, 87 gtts./min.

12) 73 ml, 90 gtts./min.   13) 47.5 ml, 93 gtts./min.

14) 6 hr.   15) 16 hr.   16) 10 hr.   17) $12\frac{1}{2}$ hr.

18) 15 gtts./min., 47 gtts./min.   19) 50 gtts./min., 40 gtts./min.

20) 25 gtts./min., 20 gtts./min.   21) 33 gtts./min., 42 gtts./min.

22) 25 gtts./min., 52 gtts./min.   23) 25 gtts./min., 32 gtts./min.

24) 100 gtts./min., 57 gtts./min.   25) 75 gtts./min., 35 gtts./min.

26) 0.75ml/min., 45 ml/hr.   27) 0.75 ml/min., 45 ml/hr.

28) 0.31 ml/min., 19 ml/hr.   29) 0.5 ml/min., 30 ml/hr.

Cumulative Review (pp. 270–279)

1) $7\frac{1}{8}$ 2) $2\frac{1}{2}$ 3) $\frac{5}{8}$ 4) $\frac{2}{5}$ 5) 2.98   6) 0.906   7) 6.698

8) $6\frac{1}{2}$ 9) $\frac{43}{8}$ 10) 20%   11) $\frac{9}{20}$ 12) 0.375   13) 83   14) 83.5

15) 83.46   16) 83.459   17) $\frac{2}{3}$ 18) 0.4%   19) 0.025   20) 18

21) 3.6   22) 16   23) 4 tabs   24) 2 oz.   25) 525 mg

26) 19.2 mg   27) 6 tabs   28) ℥ iss   29) 1.5 ℓ   30) ℥ $\frac{1}{4}$

31) ♏ x   32) gr. xv   33) 15 g   3) 2.5 mg   35) 2 tsp.

36) 2 tab.   37) 35 kg   38) 104.9°F   39) 2   40) $2\frac{1}{2}$ 41) 20

42) 450   43) $\frac{3}{4}$ 44) 5   45) 0.350   46) 7.5   47) 4   48) 0.5

49) 2   50) 30   51) 2 tab. per dose   52) 2 tab.   53) 1 tab.

54) 12 cans   55) 1.7 g   56) 145 mg   57) 0.4 ml   58) 3.3 ml

59) 2.5 ml   60) 1.5 ml   61) 0.35 ml   62) 10 ml   63) 1 ml

64) 0.6cc   65) 2.2 ml; discard   66) 1.5 ml; relabel

67) 1.25 ml; relabel   68) 100 000 U/ml, 1.5 ml   69)4.5 g or 4500 mg

70) 11.5 ml   71) 2.4 ml   72) 31 gtts./min.   73) 40 gtts./min.

74) 98 gtts./min.   75) 5.5 hr.   76) 33 gtts./min.; 43 gtts./min.

77) 150 gtts./min.   78) 106 mg   79) 256 mg   80) 800 mg per dose

81) 23 mg   82) 0.25 ml/min., 15 ml/hr.   83) 0.42 ml/min., 25 ml/hr.

Index